POST
ENDODONTIC
RESTORATION

SANDEEP DUBEY
SUSHIL LANDGE
VIKRAM BELKHODE
SEEMA MARATHE

SHWETA PANDEY
DHANASHREE CHARDE
SHARAYU V. NIMONKAR
SHAHINAWAZ S. MULANI

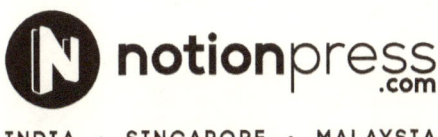

INDIA • SINGAPORE • MALAYSIA

Notion Press

Old No. 38, New No. 6
McNichols Road, Chetpet
Chennai - 600 031

First Published by Notion Press 2020
Copyright © Sandeep Dubey, Sushil Landge, Vikram Belkhode,
Seema Marathe, Sharayu V. Nimonkar, Shweta Pandey,
Dhanashree Charde, Shahinawaz S. Mulani 2020
All Rights Reserved.

ISBN 978-1-64650-750-4

This book has been published with all efforts taken to make the material error-free after the consent of the author. However, the author and the publisher do not assume and hereby disclaim any liability to any party for any loss, damage, or disruption caused by errors or omissions, whether such errors or omissions result from negligence, accident, or any other cause.

While every effort has been made to avoid any mistake or omission, this publication is being sold on the condition and understanding that neither the author nor the publishers or printers would be liable in any manner to any person by reason of any mistake or omission in this publication or for any action taken or omitted to be taken or advice rendered or accepted on the basis of this work. For any defect in printing or binding the publishers will be liable only to replace the defective copy by another copy of this work then available.

CONTENTS

Acknowledgements 5

Introduction 7

History 9

1. Altered Characteristics of Endodontically Treated Teeth 13

2. Treatment Planning 17

3. Basic Components of Postendodontic Restorations 24

4. Coronal Tooth Structure: Importance of the Ferrule 26

5. Foundation Restoration: Post and Core 29

6. Final Tooth Coverage 83

Conclusion and Summary 95

Review of Literature 97

Bibliography 107

ACKNOWLEDGEMENTS

I bow in gratitude to almighty God for giving me aptitude to endeavor this textbook. Without his blessings, I could not have completed the book.

Any textbook requires invigorating collaboration and assistance of friends, colleagues, teachers, seniors and juniors in order to complete successfully. In this regard, I would like to extend special thanks to all those who had helped to accomplish this goal.

I owe an exceptional gratitude to my teacher and mentor Dr. B. Rajkumar for his valuable support and suggestions, encouragement and blessings.

Word fail me when it comes to thanking my family members who, stand by me throughout and their encouragement helped to lighten the dark hours when inspiration failed and ideas dried up.

The excellent co-operation of the publishers is also greatly acknowledged.

INTRODUCTION

The dental practitioner is often faced with the task of restoring endodontically treated teeth. Root canal treatment is usually a consequence of dental caries followed by pulpal infection or traumatic damage to the tooth and also it is done intentionally at the time of occlusal plane correction to use the tooth as an abutment for overdentures.

Traditionally, it has been accepted that the best treatment for a posterior, endodontically-treated tooth is some form of coronal coverage. This may take the form of gold, resin composite, or amalgam restoration that covers the occlusal aspect of the tooth to prevent it from fracture. Quite a number of previously published articles and scientific papers have voiced the opinion that endodontically-treated posterior teeth (as well as anterior teeth with loss of significant coronal tooth structure) should receive crowns to protect them from fracture and extend their longevity. Crowns are not the only viable option to protect teeth following obturation. Cuspal coverage may also be provided by complex amalgams and by gold, ceramic, and resin composite onlays.

Trauma and decay are mostly associated with an extensive loss of tooth structure, necessitating restoration of the tooth with a complete crown for esthetic and functional rehabilitation. When a large portion of the crown has been lost to damage it is often impossible to achieve sufficient anchorage of restoration in the remaining dentin. In such situations, root canal-retained restoration is required.

Opinions on the restoration of root-filled teeth are mainly based on empirical data, which claim that a root-filled tooth is more fragile than a vital one and thus needs to be reinforced with a post to minimize the risk of root fracture.

Posts and cores in endodontically treated teeth have been utilized for more than a century as a means to retain the foundation of the final restoration. However, it has been shown, that they can weaken the tooth. Failures of traditional metal post restorations are caused mainly by root canal fracture due to the very different modulus of elasticity of the tooth structure and metal post. Custom cast metal posts and cores used to retain restorations remain indicated only in endodontically treated teeth with small clinical crowns. Metal posts are not indicated for people with metal allergies. The range of indications for a cast metal post and core system as an indirect prosthodontic procedure has recently become smaller, indeed. Nowadays, metal free posts have been introduced for post and core endodontic restorations. Their dramatically different physical properties allow them to dissipate compressive, tensile and shear stress, rather than transferring and concentrating excessive loading in the residual root structures as with metal posts.

HISTORY

Past is history—is a common saying in English, but the question is "can we forget the past or rather should we forget the past?" for this question Winston Churchill's phrase is an apt reply. He said, *"The longer u can look back, the further u can look forward".* It is a fact that one cannot fully evaluate the problems of the present without knowing the past. The same is true with dentistry. The past is recalled here in a spirit of humility to inspire the future.

The newspaper headline read—"Ancient root canal filling found". Datelined Jerusalem the article went on to state that " A green tooth containing the oldest known root canal filling was discovered in the skull of a Nabatean warrior who was buried in a mass grave 2200 years ago. The tooth in question dated from the Hellenistic period (200 BC). Radiographic examination of this skull showed a 2.5mm bronze wire that had been implanted in the root canal – the earliest known archeological example of a tooth filled with a metal object." Professor Jias explain that this was the probable reason for *'primitive endodontics'.* [19]

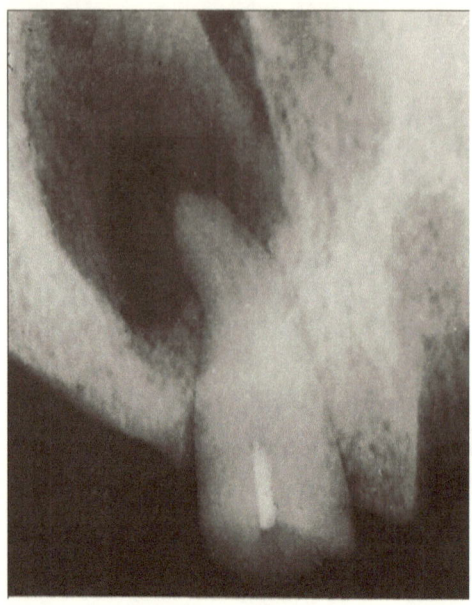

Various methods of restoring pulpless teeth have been reported for more than 200 years. In *1747*, **Pierre Fauchard** described the process by which the roots of maxillary anterior teeth were used for the restoration of single teeth and the replacement of multiple teeth. Posts were fabricated of gold and silver and held in the root canal space with a heat softened adhesive called *"mastic"* prepared by gum, lac, turpentine, and white coral powder. The longevity of the restorations made using the technique was attested to by Fauchard: "Teeth and artificial dentures, fastened with posts and gold wires, hold better than all others. They sometimes last fifteen to twenty years and even more without displacement. Common thread and silk, used ordinarily to attach all kinds of teeth or artificial pieces, do not last long".[19]

Back in early 19th century the Replacement crowns were made from bone, ivory, animal teeth, and sound natural tooth crowns. Gradually, the use of these natural substances declined, to be slowly replaced by porcelain. A *pivot* (what today is termed as a post) was used to retain the artificial porcelain crown into a root canal, and the crown post combination was termed as *"pivot crown"*. Porcelain pivot crowns were described by a dentist in Paris, **Dubois de Chemant.** Pivoting of artificial crowns to natural roots became the most common method of replacing artificial teeth and was reported to be the "best that can be employed" by *Chapin Harris in The Dental Art in 1839.* [19]

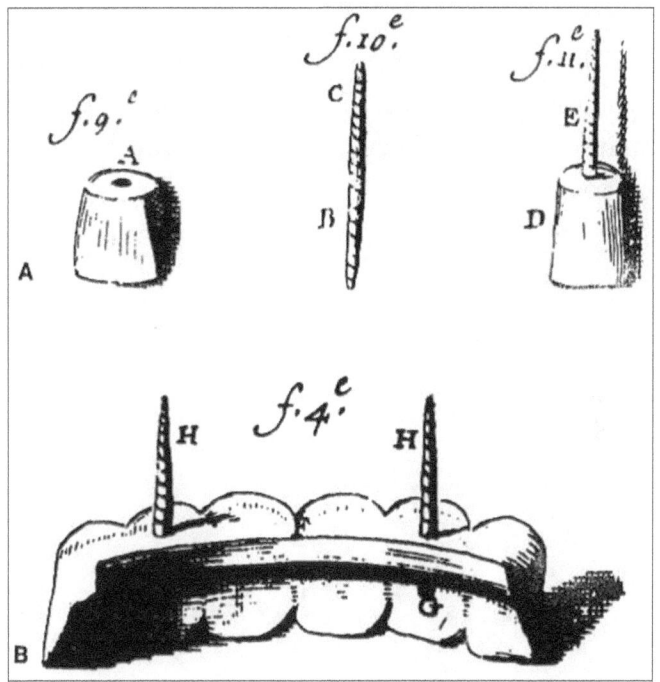

Early pivot crowns in the United States used seasoned wood (white hickory) pivots. The pivot was adapted to the inside surface of an all-ceramic crown and also into the root canal space. Moisture would swell the wood and retain the pivot in place. Subsequently, pivot crowns were fabricated using wood/metal combinations. And then more durable all-metal pivots were used. Metal pivot retention was achieved by various means such as threads, pins, surface roughening and split designs that provided mechanical spring retention.

Unfortunatly, cement that would have increased post retention and decreased abrasion of the root caused by the movement of metal posts within the root canals were not used. Endodontic therapy by these dental pioneers embraced only minimal efforts to clean shape and obturate the canals.

Frequent use of wood posts led to repeated episodes of swelling and pain. Wood posts, however, did not allow the escape of the so-called *"morbid-humors"*.[19] A groove in the post or root canal provided a pathway for continual suppuration from the peri radicular tissues.

Today both the endodontic and prosthodontic aspects of treatment have advanced significantly. New materials and techniques have been developed, and a substantial body of knowledge is available on which clinical treatment decisions are based.

ALTERED CHARACTERISTICS OF ENDODONTICALLY TREATED TEETH

Restoration of endodontically treated teeth replace missing tooth structure, maintains function and esthetics, and protects against fracture and infection. Successful endodontic debridement and apical sealing are essential underpinnings for the restoration of the nonvital tooth. With improved and advanced endodontic techniques, the well-treated pulpless tooth can very well function as an integral part of the dental apparatus as long as it is adequately restored. [20]

Endodontically treated teeth are structurally different from unrestored vital teeth and require specialized restorative treatment.

The various changes in a root canal treated tooth include

1. Loss of tooth structure.
2. Altered physical characteristics.
3. Altered esthetic characteristics.

LOSS OF TOOTH STRUCTURE

- ❖ The diminished volume of the tooth structure from the combined effects of previous disease, dental procedure, and endodontic therapy, significantly weakens nonvital teeth.
- ❖ Endodontic access to the pulp chamber destroys the structural integrity provided by the coronal dentin of the pulpal ceiling allowing greater flexion of the tooth under function.

- Also, accidental penitration through the pulpal floor creates an open conduit between the oral cavity and the alveolar bone which must be prevented by careful access preparation and if it occurs then it must be sealed to prevent the ingress of bacteria.
- This reduction in tooth strength is primarily due to loss of coronal tooth structure and less because of instrumentation within the canal. *[root canal procedures reduce the stiffness of the tooth only by 5%, whereas tooth structure removal in mesio-occluso-distal preparation reduces it by 60%]*.[8,20]

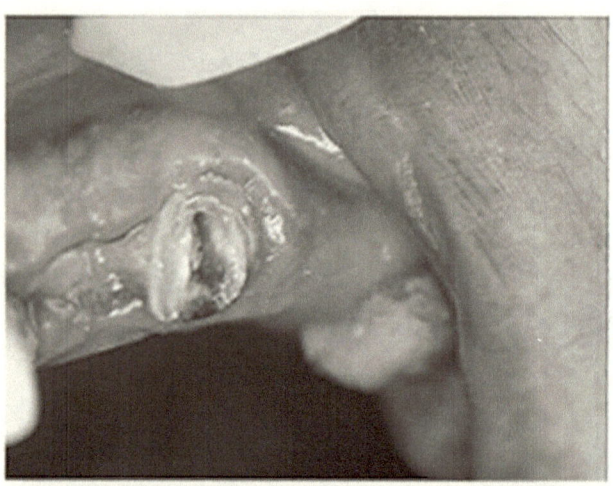

ALTERED PHYSICAL CHARACTERISTICS

The tooth structure remaining after endodontic treatment shows irreversible altered physical characteristics.

- Changes in collagen cross-linking and dehydration of the dentin results in a 14% reduction in strength and toughness.
- There is no blood supply to the tooth, the dentin permeability decreases and since the pulp is not present there is no secondary dentin formation and the tooth become more prone to fracture.
- Maxillary teeth are stronger than mandibular teeth, with mandibular incisors being the weakest.

- ❖ The combined loss of structural integrity, loss of moisture and loss of dentin toughness compromises endodontically treated teeth and necessitates special care during restoration. [20]

ALTERED ESTHETIC CHARACTERISTICS

- ❖ The darkening of the nonvital teeth is a common clinical finding. Biochemically altered dentin modifies light refraction through the tooth and correspondingly modifies its appearance.
- ❖ Inadequate cleaning and shaping of the root canals can leave vital tissue in the coronal pulp horns, which upon disintegration results in tooth darkening.
- ❖ The chief objective is to restore a tooth with an esthetic restoration that is both biologically and mechanically sound. This relies on creating adequate resistance and retention form and also reinforcement and replacement of remaining tooth structure. [8]

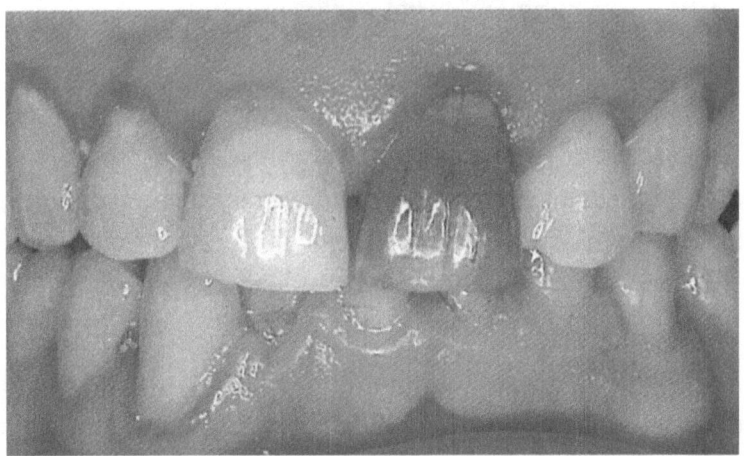

PHILOSOPHY OF PREPARATION

Endodontic treatment removes the vital contents of the canal, leaving the tooth pulpless and resulting in teeth with calcified tissues that contain significantly less moisture than that of vital teeth. Therefore it is imperative that absolute preoperative planning and extreme care must be utilized in the selection of the type and design of the final coronal restoration, once the endodontic therapy is completed satisfactorily.[13]

TIMING THE RESTORATIVE PROCEDURE

Endodontic treatment must be a part of an overall strategy for the treatment of the patient. It may be better to consider extraction and construction of a fixed prosthesis when the condition of the tooth to be root canal treated makes it unrestorable.[17]

However once the decision to perform root canal treatment is taken, the question that arises is – How long to wait before placing the final restoration?

The following factors are to be considered for the above mentioned question:-

1. The pre existing endodontic status.
2. The quality of the root canal filling.
3. The site of the tooth in the mouth.
4. The type of restoration to be placed.

Given a satisfactory technical result on the final radiograph of the treated tooth and in the absence of symptoms, where the pulp had previously been vital, it would be reasonable to proceed immediately to the placement of the final restoration.

In contrast, if there has been an apical radiolucency before treatment associated with an unsatisfactory root canal filling, it would be sensible to delay the final restoration until evidence of periradicular healing is seen radiographically.[17]

During this time, the remaining tooth structure should be protected by an adequate interim restoration which must also be capable of preventing coronal leakage that would otherwise adversely influence the outcome.

TREATMENT PLANNING

When the decision is made to treat the tooth endodontically, consideration must be given to its subsequent restoration.

Existing endodontically treated teeth need to be assessed carefully for the following:- [32]

1. Good apical seal.
2. No exudates.
3. No fistula.
4. Absence of active inflammation.
5. No apical sensitivity.
6. No sensitivity to pressure.
7. Radiographic examination.

Inadequate root fillings should be retreated and, in case of a doubt, the tooth monitored till the symptoms subside.

All changes that accompany the root canal therapy influence the selection of the restorative materials and procedures for endodontically treated teeth. [20]

Important considerations include the following:-

1. The amount of tooth structure remaining.
2. The anatomic position of the tooth.
3. The occlusal forces on the tooth.
4. The restorative requirements of the tooth.
5. The esthetic requirements of the tooth.

ANTERIOR TEETH

It can be restored using either:- [29]

- ❖ Composite resins.
- ❖ Glass ionomer cement.
- ❖ Laminates and Veneers.

In extensively damaged teeth:-

- ❖ Three-quarter crown.
- ❖ Porcelain jacket crown.

Conservative restoration of anterior teeth

- ❖ Anterior teeth do not always need complete coverage, except when plastic restorative materials would have limited prognosis in view of the extent of coronal destruction. Although commonly believed, it has not been demonstrated experimentally that endodontically treated teeth are weaker or more brittle than vital teeth. However their moisture content may be reduced. [Study was done by Helfer AR, et al]. [32]
- ❖ Laboratory testing has revealed a similar resistance to fracture between untreated and endodontically treated anterior teeth.
- ❖ In anterior teeth where there has been little previous tooth destruction. Restoration may be done using a combination of composite resin placed over a base of glass ionomer cement.
- ❖ Composite resin is the most appropriate material for restoring the access cavity, given its physical properties and a high quality surface finish, together with a good seal achieved by acid-etching enamel.
- ❖ Care must be taken to ensure that the root canal filling is removed from the crown of the tooth if discoloration of the dentin due to endodontic sealers containing eugenol is to be prevented. To prevent discoloration, a sitting for intra coronal etching with superoxol is done before filling the pulp chamber after root canal obturation.

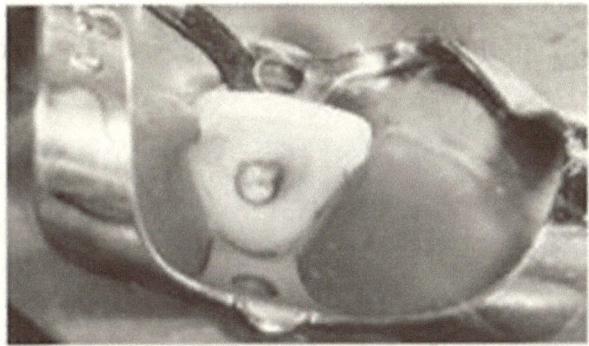

❖ Fractured crowns of anterior teeth can be restored using *cemented pins*. Grooves are prepared in the remaining tooth structure for the pins and the tooth is built up.

Tooth reinforcement

There is no indication for the placement of a post with in the root canal of a relatively intact anterior tooth. Placing a post in an endodontically treated tooth is a fairly common practice despite the paucity of data to support its success. In fact, a laboratory study and two stress analyses have determined that no significant reinforcement results. This might be explained by the hypothesis that, when the tooth is loaded, stresses are greatest at the facial and lingual surfaces of the root and an internal post being only minimally stressed does not help in preventing fracture. [17]

In addition, there are disadvantages to the routine use of a cemented post:-

1. Placing a post requires additional restorative procedures.
2. Preparing a tooth to accommodate the post removes additional tooth structure.
3. It may be difficult to restore a tooth later, when a complete crown is needed, because the cemented post may have failed to provide adequate retention for the core material.
4. The post can complicate or prevent future endodontic retreatment if it becomes necessary.

Discoloration in the absence of significant loss of tooth structure may be better treated by *bleaching*. It is not usually done because a number of studies have indicated the possible dangers of resorption following bleaching.[8]

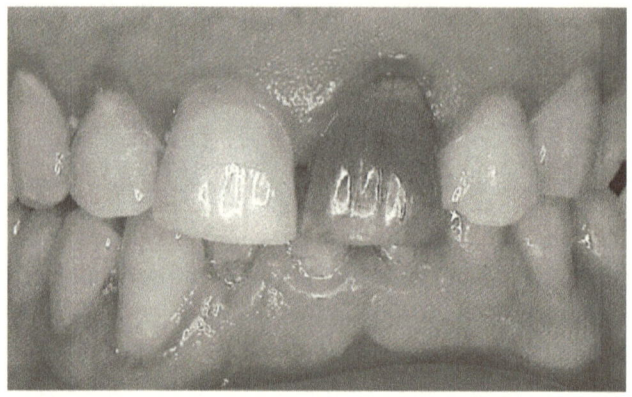

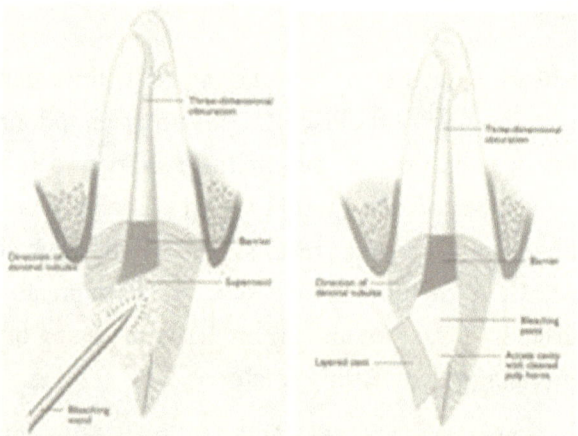

Anterior crowns without post

1. There are times when a crown is necessary for a root canal treated anterior tooth. But it is certainly not necessary that in these instances the tooth will require placement of a post. Maxillary incisors are wide at the cemento-enamel junction.

2. When the access cavity is prepared properly there is usually enough coronal structure remaining to allow the dentine core to support the

crown without the need to place a post after tooth preparation. This can also be achieved by making access to the pulp chamber through the incisal edge or just palatal to it, so that more amount of palatal dentine remains intact. [17]

3. The labio lingual dimension of the mandibular incisors at the junction between the crown and the root is small; combination of the loss of tooth structure produced by the endodontic access cavity and the crown preparation generally removes a large amount of tooth structure which necessitates the placement of a post.

POSTERIOR TEETH

It can be restored using:- [29]

- Amalgam restoration.
- Adhesive restorations i.e. composites.[for esthetics]
- Onlay covering one or more cusps.
- Full crown.

Endodontically treated posterior teeth are subjected to more occlusal loading than their anterior counterparts because of their position closer to the insertion of the masticatory muscles. This combined with their morphologic characteristics, makes them more susceptible to fracture. Careful occlusal adjustment will reduce potentially damaging lateral forces during excursive jaw movements, but it is suggested that any endodontically treated posterior tooth receive cuspal coverage to prevent biting forces from wedging the cusps apart. [20]

Adhesive restorations for posterior teeth

1. The endodontic access cavity in a posterior tooth not only removes the roof of the pulp chamber but also creates a wide occlusal isthmus. Consequently, even if both the marginal ridges remain intact, the tooth is at some risk of fracture.

2. The reason for choosing this restorative material is mainly the esthetic concern of the patient, and is used mainly for the premolars.
3. The other alternative to this restoration is a ceramic crown. These restorations are only used if the material is durably and effectively bonded to the dental tissues by means of an acid etch enamel technique, perhaps enhanced by dentin bonding. The effect of polymerization shrinkage that it induces stresses within the adjacent tooth structure thereby producing cuspal displacement.
4. From an occlusal standpoint, such composite restorations present problems when large because the ultimate shaping and finishing of the occlusal surface have to be carried out with rotary instruments. Trying to produce precise occlusal functional form by such means is unlikely to be successful. Though it can be argued that in smaller sized cavities on the occlusal surface of posterior teeth composites present as a good option.
5. Another factor affecting stability in the occlusion will be the resistance of the composite to wear and also its effect on the wear of opposing teeth.

Indirect tooth colored adhesive restorations

1. The introduction of indirect posterior composite restorations was intended to address many of the above mentioned problems.
2. The effect of polymerization shrinkage on the tooth structure is virtually eliminated by employing an indirect technique, and restorations can be made with accurate occlusal contacts. However they are expensive and compared with conventional techniques for gold and porcelain restoration, the precision of fit is disappointing.
3. Any strengthening effect from these restorations will be reliant on the stability of the composite luting agent.
4. Ceramic inlays are another alternative. The long term performance of such restorations particularly in endodontically treated teeth is yet unknown. However there does appear to be a growing agreement that,

where the isthmus is large, onlay, rather than inlay, construction is preferred for both composite resin and ceramic restorations.

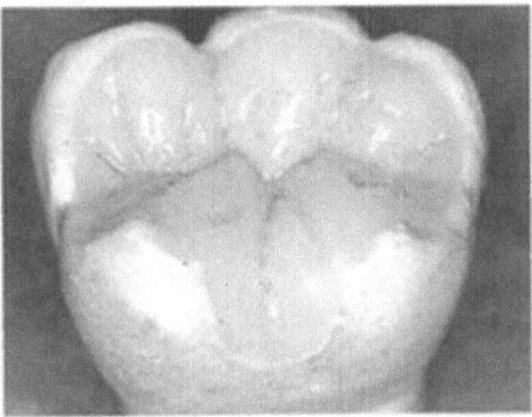

It is difficult to achieve an amalgam restoration which has a good combination of cuspal coverage and proper occlusal form.

Two things can be concluded:-

- ❖ Cuspal coverage is necessary to minimize the possibility of fracture.
- ❖ Onlay restorations in cast metal are more likely to have a long term occlusal stability than those made from composite resin or ceramic.

BASIC COMPONENTS OF POSTENDODONTIC RESTORATIONS

Restorations for endodontically treated teeth are designed to:
1. Protect the remaining tooth from fracture.
2. Prevent reinfection of the root canal system.
3. Replace the missing tooth structure.

Basic components are:

a. Residual coronal and radicular tooth structure supported by the periodontium.
b. The post: Located in the root and it retains the core.
c. The core: Located in the pulp chamber and coronal area of the tooth and it replaces the missing crown structure.
d. Coronal restoration: Protects the tooth and restores function and esthetics. [20]

All these components are joined together by the adhesive bonding agents or luting cements.

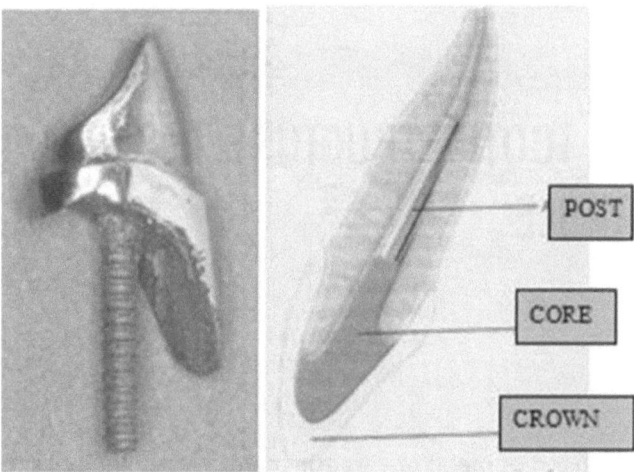

The selection for the individual components of the restoration depends on:-

a. Location of the root.
b. Functional requirements of the tooth.
c. The amount of missing coronal or radicular tooth structure.

CORONAL TOOTH STRUCTURE: IMPORTANCE OF THE FERRULE

Ferrule: It is a band of metal or ceramic material that encircles the external dimension of the residual tooth similar to the metal bands around a barrel or a shovel handle. It is given to prevent fracture of the roots. It is formed by the walls and the margins of the crown or by cast telescopic coping encasing at least 2 to 3 mm of sound tooth structure. [8, 19, 20]

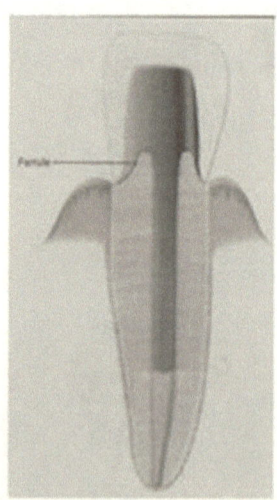

IDEAL REQUIREMENTS

1. The dentin axial wall height should be at least 2 to 3 mm.
2. The axial walls must be parallel.

3. The restoration must completely encircle the tooth.
4. The margin must be on solid and sound tooth structure.
5. The crown and crown preparation must not invade the attachment apparatus. [20]

A properly executed ferrule significantly reduces the incidence of fracture in a non vital tooth by reinforcing the tooth at its external surface and dissipating force that concentrates at the narrowest circumference of the tooth. A longer ferrule increases the fracture resistance and also resists the lateral forces from posts and leverage form crown in function and increases the retention and resistance of the restoration. [35]

Once the crown is fitted on a tooth having a ferrule prepared on it, the lateral forces transmitted from the crown to the post result in compression of the dentin coronally and it does not put the dentin and the post under tension. This is known as the *ferrule effect.* [20, 35]

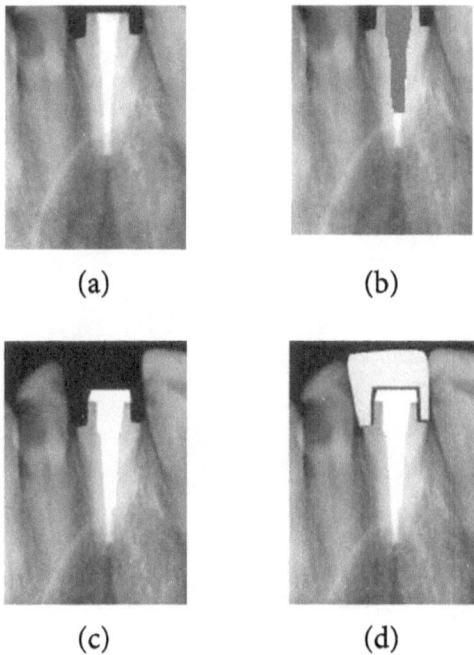

(a)　　　　　(b)

(c)　　　　　(d)

This means that a 4 to 5 mm height and 1 mm thickness of sound, suprabony tooth structure should be available to accommodate both the periodontal and biologic width of the ferrule. A tooth lacking sufficient structure for a ferrule must be evaluated for periodontal crown lengthening surgery for crown elongation or orthodontic extrusion to gain access to additional root surface. The lack of proper ferrule in final restoration forces the core and the dowel to accept high functional stresses, often resulting in fracture caused by material failure.

FOUNDATION RESTORATION: POST AND CORE

The post, the core and their luting or bonding agents together form a *foundation restoration* to support a coronal restoration for the endodontically treated tooth. [20]

POST

It is a restorative dental material that is placed in the root of a structurally damaged tooth in which additional retention is needed for the core and the coronal restoration. [20]

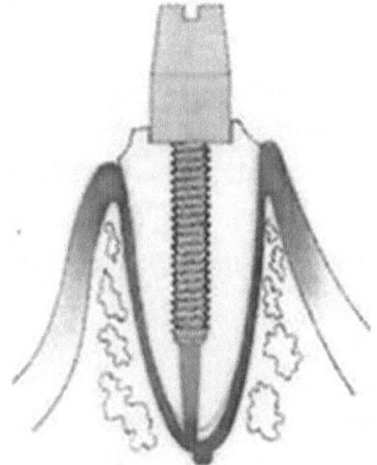

It is used when coronal structure is missing more than 2 proximal surfaces along with 1 axial wall.

It is either cemented or threaded into a prepared channel to retain the restoration and to protect the remaining tooth structure.

Posts transmit occlusal forces or masticatory forces favorably to the remaining root structure and periodontium.

Posts should provide the following clinical features:-

1. *Maximal protection of the root from fracture:* It should be remembered that post itself does not strengthen or reinforce the tooth. Dentin should not be sacrificed to place a large post in teeth with little tooth structure remaining as this dentin along with the surrounding alveolar bone provides strength to the tooth.
2. *Maximum retention within the root and retrievability.*
3. *Maximal retention of the core and crown:* The post should extend coronally from the root to anchor the core and subsequently the crown.
4. *Maximal protection of the crowns' marginal seal from coronal leakage:* This occurs due to bacterial contamination.
5. *Pleasing esthetics where indicated:* In the esthetic zone the post should not detract from the esthetics of the coronal tooth structure, ceramic crown or gingiva. Current restorative procedures allow fabrication of highly esthetic ceramic coronal restorations that have no metal substructure. These restorations have remarkable depth of life like color and vitality with no unnatural opacity, shadows, gray coloration, or artificial brightness from underlying metal or metal masking agents.
6. *High radiographic visibility.*
7. *Bio compatibility.*

An ideal post should have an optimal combination *of resilience, stiffness, flexibility and strength.* [19, 20]

- It should be resilient enough to cushion an impact by stretching elastically, thereby reducing the stress to the root.
- It should return to its normal shape without permanent deformation.

SELECTION OF POSTS

How well a specific post functions in the tooth depends on the stiffness/flexibility of the post, the amount of remaining tooth structure, the lateral forces the post and tooth complex must withstand, and the fatigue strength of the post.

Occlusal forces, bruxism, anterior guidance, and sudden traumatic impact all affect the teeth and endodontic posts.

Current post systems are designed to provide the best compromise between the desired properties and the inherent limitations of the available materials.

CLASSIFICATION OF POSTS

Type of material used

a. Rigid
a. Non rigid

Method of fabrication

a. Custom made
b. Prefabricated
    * Threaded posts
    * Cemented posts

According to walter

Prefabricated posts

a. *Active:* Active posts are threaded and are intended to engage the walls of the canal.
    i. *Tapered self threaded post systems:* They are screwed into a channel prepared with matched reamers. An example is Dentatus screw.[13]

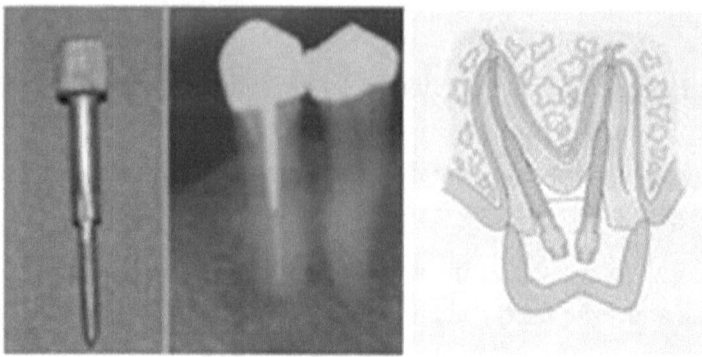

ii. **Parallel sided, threaded post systems:** They engage the dentin wall by self threading or with use of matched taps. Examples are the Radix Anchor which is self taped, and the Kurer Anchor which is first tapped and then threaded into the dentin.[13]

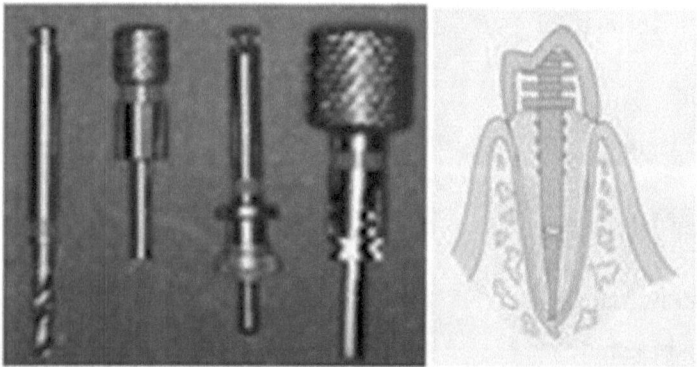

b. **Passive:** Passive posts are retained only by the luting agents.
   i. ***Tapered smooth sided post systems:*** They are cemented into a channel prepared with endodontic files or reamers of matching sizes. An example is the Kerr Endopost. [Cemented posts]. [13]

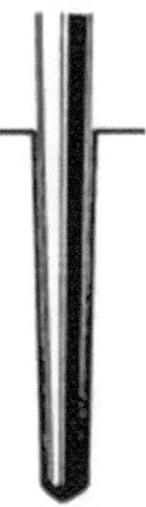

   ii. ***Parallel sided, serrated and vented post systems:*** They are cemented into a matched channel prepared with a twist drill of matching size.[8] An example is the Whaledent's Parapost system.

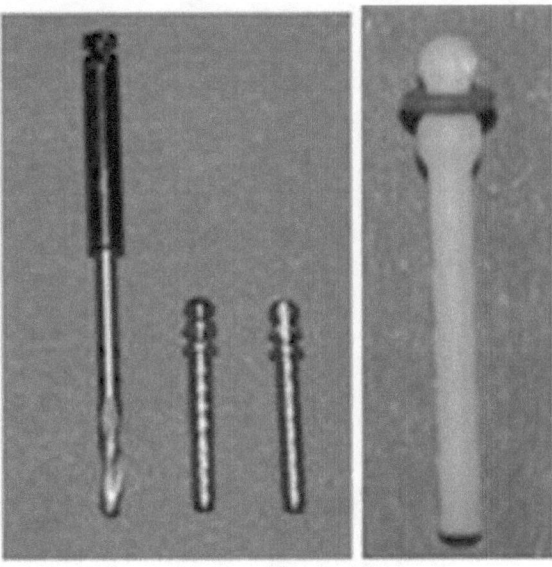

iii. *Parallel with tapered apical end.*

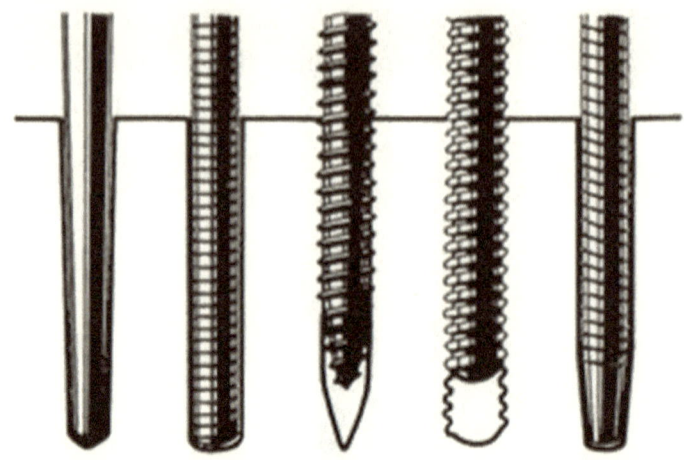

Various designs and shapes of posts are available. They are:- [29]

- ❖ Tapered smooth posts.
- ❖ Tapered threaded screw type posts.
- ❖ Parallel sided serrated posts.
- ❖ Parallel sided tapered end posts.
- ❖ Parallel sided threaded posts.
- ❖ Tapered notch type posts.
- ❖ Splitted tapered self threaded screw type posts.
- ❖ Parallel sided notched surface.
- ❖ Parallel sided with tapered end and notched surface posts.
- ❖ Splitted parallel sided threaded screw type posts.

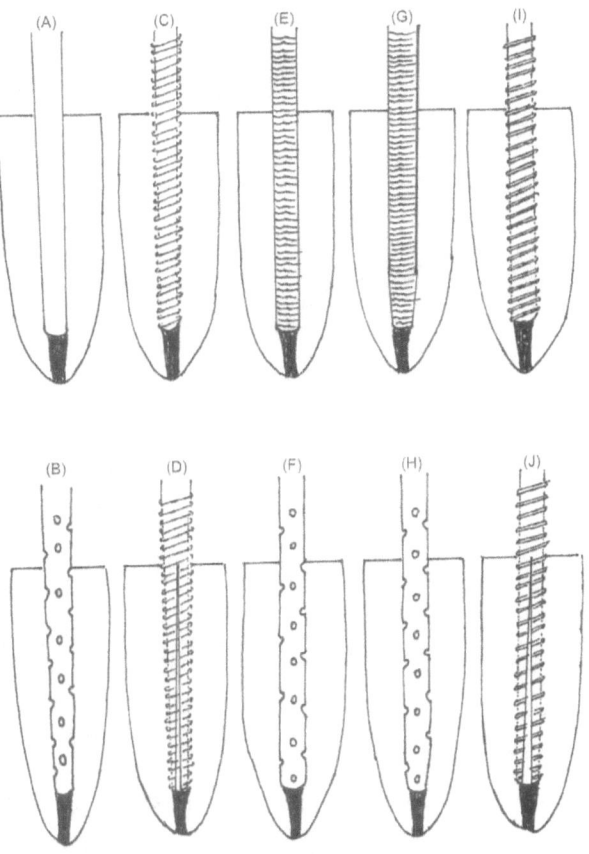

Rigid post systems

Traditionally, posts which have along clinical history were metal and were either custom cast or preformed. Metallic posts include crown and bridge alloys, stainless steel, or titanium alloy.

- ❖ Zirconia posts are esthetic, adhesive and very rigid but also brittle alternatives to metal. These posts are very hard and cannot be cut from the canal this creates a problem if retreatment needs to be done.

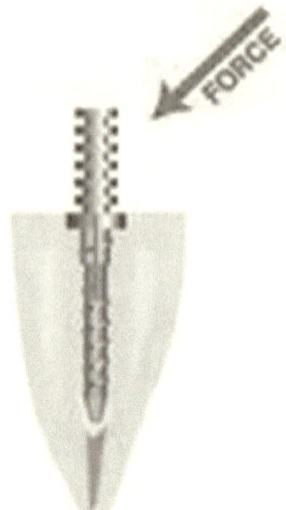

- Titanium, gold and zirconia posts are biocompatible. But stainless steel posts contain nickel, an allergen that can leach out through dentin tubules into the tissues.
- The color and opacity of metal posts can interfere with esthetic restorations.
- Amongst rigid posts, zirconia is the stiffest. Stainless steel is tougher than titanium alloy, which is stiffer than pure titanium.
- Cast gold, stainless steel, and zirconia posts are all radio opaque are easily visible on the radiographs. The radioopacity of titanium posts is similar to guttapercha. [20]
- These posts prevent tooth fracture by dissipating functional forces along the length of the root and the periodontal structures.

Non rigid post systems

- Non rigid posts are biocompatible and are composed of glass, quartz or carbon fibers embedded in a resin matrix. These posts are designed to have physical properties similar to dentin. Glass and quartz fiber posts are translucent or white; these esthetic options enhance esthetic restorations.

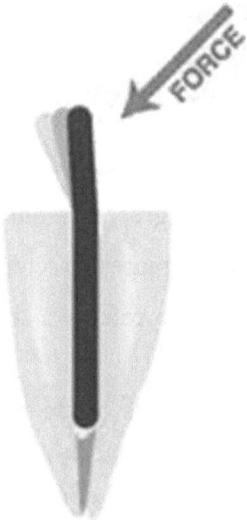

- In structurally sound teeth these posts flex with the tooth under functional forces, thus reducing the transfer of force to the root and reducing the risk of root fracture. [20]
- The primary benefit of resilient posts with a lower modulus of elasticity is protection of the root from fracture through reduction of transfer of forces from post to root. This post flexibility is beneficial for teeth with more than 3-4 mm of remaining axial dentin which provides cervical stiffness to the tooth/post/core complex. These posts are not of much use in severely destructed teeth as it has been observed that—since these posts have the same modulus of elasticity as root but is much thinner in diameter, it will flex more under load. This can cause leakage under the crown buildup along with movement of the post which can cause micro movement of the core, disruption of the cement seal, loss of core or crown.

POST SIZE, POST SPACE AND ROOT ANATOMY

The post should be long enough to satisfy the clinical requirements without jeopardizing the apical seal or risking perforation of a narrowing or fluted root. It should be as long as possible, conform to the shape of the root canal, lie within the long axis of the tooth and be of a minimum diameter to maximize preservation of remaining dentin.

Many clinical studies on retention of posts have shown that:-

1. The longer the post, the greater is the retention.
2. Parallel sided posts have greater retention that tapered posts.
3. Roughening the post increases its retention.
4. Threaded posts are more retentive than posts with other surface finishes.
5. Increased post length leads to decreased stress. A reduction of compression and shear concentrations occurs with increased post height. Accompanying the increased reduction in stress is an increased resistance to fracture. The longer the post, the greater is the retention and support and better is the stress distribution. Short posts are dangerous and often lead to fracture of the tooth because they are not completely surrounded by periradicular bone. Also the fulcrum point of a short post is closer to the occlusal table and may not be located in the area of the root supported within the alveolar bone.

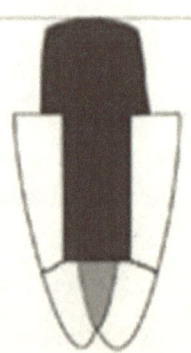

6 At the very least the post should be equal the length of the clinical crown.

The greatest advantage of the prefabricated post systems is their ability to provide long posts to gain the important properties of retention and stress distribution.

Root morphology also affects the length and placement of posts. Root curvature reduces post length. Greater the curve of the root and more coronally placed curve, shorter is the post that is used. [20]

Despite recommendation for 1 mm of remaining dentin in post preparation procedures, the dentine thickness in the furcation of mandibular molars has been reported to be less than 1 mm in 82% of teeth. Preparation with No. 4 Gates-Glidden drill resulted in strip perforations of the furcal surface of 7.3% of the teeth; less than 0.5 mm of dentin thickness remained in 40% of the teeth. Post space drills larger than No.3 Gates-Glidden drill should not be used in distal root of mandibular molars. [20]

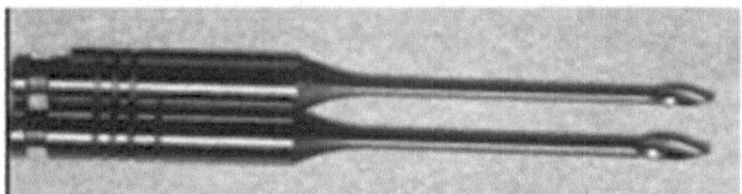

Multi rooted teeth

Root anatomy of multi rooted teeth makes it suitable to place a post in:-

- ❖ Palatal canal of maxillary molars.
- ❖ Palatal roots of maxillary premolars
- ❖ Distal roots of mandibular molars.

RETENTION OF POST TO THE ROOT

Post *cementation* and retention in the root is a critical factor in the longevity of prosthetic restorations. Factors affecting post retention are:

i. The cement used.
ii. The post material.
iii. The surface texture.
iv. Operator technique.

v. The post length.

vi. Amount of remaining tooth structure.

- ❖ Ideally retention of all types of posts is affected by the cement selection. The type of cement mainly affects the retention of tapered smooth sided posts. Traditional cements example zinc phosphate cements being most retentive and carboxylate cements exhibiting intermediate retention. These cements provide retention by mechanical means any do not have any chemical bond to the dentin or post. The lack of chemical bond becomes advantageous if removal of the post becomes necessary.

- ❖ Resin modified glass ionomer cements are not used for cementation as these cements show hygroscopic expansion, which can lead to root fracture.

- ❖ The objective of cementation is to lute a post in place with minimum film thickness between the dentin and the post. Vertical vents in the post design reduce hydrostatic back pressures that build up during cementation and reduce film thickness. Minimum film thickness is obtained with parallel sided vented posts. [8]

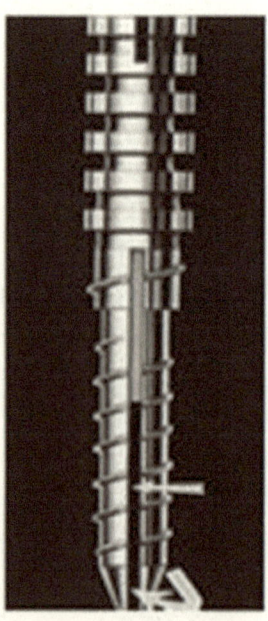

- Post cementation using unfilled BIS-GMA resins offers Better reasults. Bonded cements show less microleakage than traditional cements. Complete sealing of apical third is desirable to protect the apical seal from potential coronal microleakage.
- Greater tensile and shear forces are needed to unseat restorations placed with luting agents having higher compressive strengths. Unfilled BIS-GMA resins have compressive strengths that are approximately 2½ times greater than luting agents meeting the ADA specification no.8 [for compressive strengths of cements].[20]
- Adhesion of cementing agents is more important that their resistance to shearing forces and this can be increased by eliminating the smear layer prior to cementation and by using unfilled resins.

Disadvantages

a. Residual gutta-percha, smear layer, debris and sealer embaded on the canal wall in the dentinal tubules reduces the bonding area.

b. Cement placed on a post can trap air at the apical end of the canal and escaping air bubbles leave voids in the cement.

c. Placement of resin cement in the canal can result in premature setting because of acceleration from the bonding agent, thereby preventing seating of post.

Dentin, resin cement, post and core together are often described as forming a strong *foundation restoration*, with the adhesive cement being the unifying bond between the components. [20]

FAILURES OF CEMENTATION

a. Failure of the adhesive bonding of the post in the dentin results in debonding failures of the restoration. This is seen more often in fiber posts.

b. Marginal integrity of a dislodged and recemented post and core cannot be ensured.
c. There is a chance of recontamination of the post space through coronal leakage before the final restoration is inserted and this contamination increases the longer the post space remains empty.

To prevent this, the pulp chamber should be sealed with cotton and a maximum amount of temporary filling to resist leakage.

RETENTION OF THE POST TO THE CORE

- The post's ability to anchor the core is critically important for the sucessful reconstruction of an endodontically treated tooth.
- Loss of core retention results in loss of crown.
- In the experimental pull out tests, metal posts were more fracture resistant and therefore more retentive than carbon fiber posts.
- In vitro studies have shown that titanium posts are more retentive than glass fiber posts, which were more retentive than ceramic posts.
- Stainless steel posts were more retentive to composite cores than carbon fiber posts.
- Sharply textured titanium posts are more retentive to composite than those with rounded texture.
- Posts designed with mechanical locking features in the heads and roughened surface texture can show better retention of the core. Although a large, retentive post is beneficial for a large tooth and core, in a small anterior tooth a large post head can occupy most of the space available for the crown preparation which results in a thin layer of crown build up that leads to tooth fracture. [20]

THE COMPOSITION OF POSTS AND CORES

- Fiber and zirconia posts chemically bond to composite resin core materials. A post that retains a core of another material however is at a risk for separation of post from the core; more so in damaged teeth.

- Integrated post core systems in which the post and core is formed simultaneously from the same material eliminate this interface. These are traditionally custom cast metal cores but they can include zirconia/ceramic cores. These cores are at a risk for fracture as a result of potential casting porosity at the junction of the large core and narrow post.

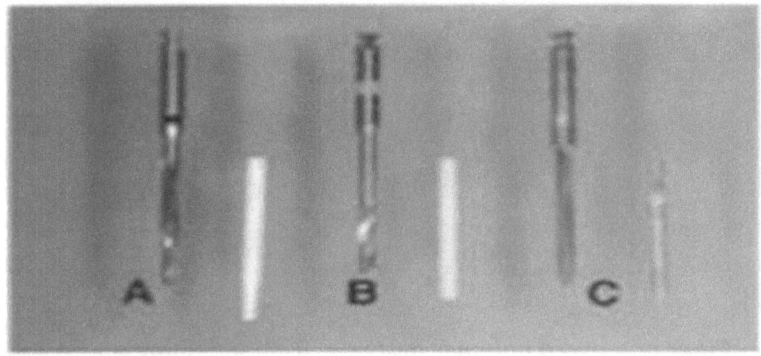

A: Zirconia posts.
B: Fiber reinforced composite posts.
C: Titanium posts

RECENT ADVANCES IN POSTS

Recently, posts made of following materials have been introduced:-

- *Carbon fiber* e.g. C-Post, Aesthetic Post, Light Post. 19,[35]
- These posts are made up of unidirectional carbon fibers embedded in an epoxy matrix. These posts possess adequate rigidity and are not prone to produce root fracture. It is shown in studies that carbon posts can be removed from the teeth as well. Carbon fiber posts are black and can reflect through gingiva, tooth structure or ceramic restorations. These posts are appropriate for teeth to be restored with gold, porcelain fused to metal crowns. Esthetic versions of this post have a quartz exterior that makes the post tooth colored.

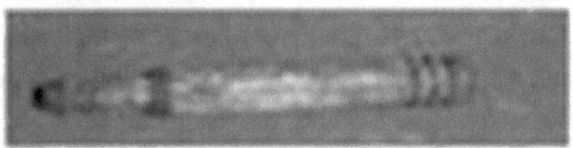

- *Ceramic material* e.g. Cerapost, Cosmopost.[35]

    These posts are made from zirconium dioxide. These posts have very high flexural strength and are very hard.

    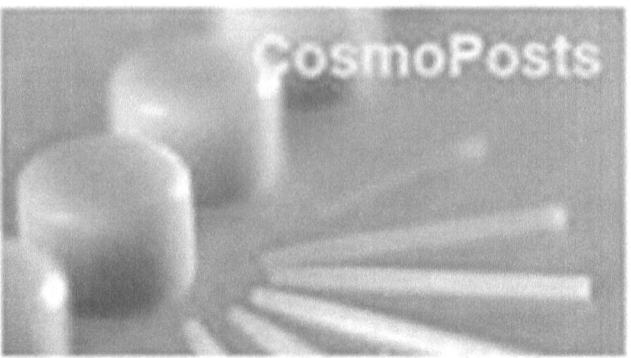

- *Fiber reinforced polymer posts* e.g. Ribbond, Fibrekor Post System, Snow post. 19,[35]

    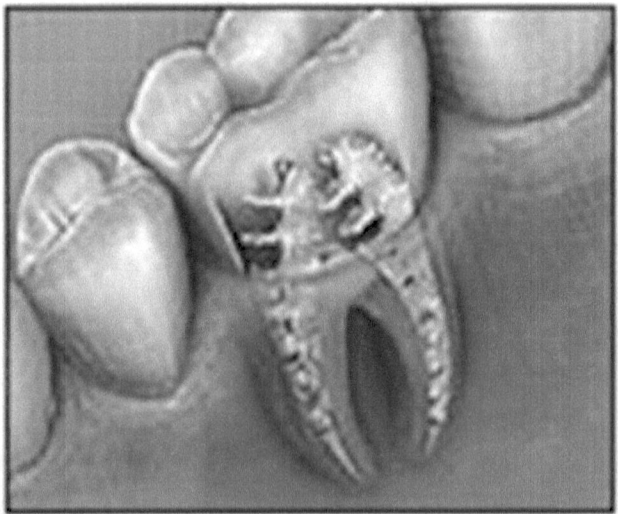

    the post have modulus of elasticity less than or equal to dentin (18 GPa). The present invention is preferably made of medical grade optical glass fibers or fiberglass fibers. The microfilaments of the present invention are treated to impart flexibility to each fiber. The fibers are twisted by twisting on other non axial arrangements of fibers to impart strength to the unit post. This allows it to function as a permanent post in the tooth. These posts are made up of woven polyethylene fiber ribbon that is coated with a dentin bonding agent and is packed into the canal, where it is then light polymerized in position.

These posts have been shown to reinforce weak teeth with flared canals. They do not require additional tooth preparation as they conform to the shape of the canal; therefore they preserve the integrity of the canal. These posts can be easily retrieved from the canal if need arises. A fiberglass post behaves like a *mono block*. All the forces acting on this post are equally distributed to the periodontium thereby reducing risk of fracture. These posts reduced the incidence of vertical root fracture.

❖ *Light post* e.g. DT light post system. 35

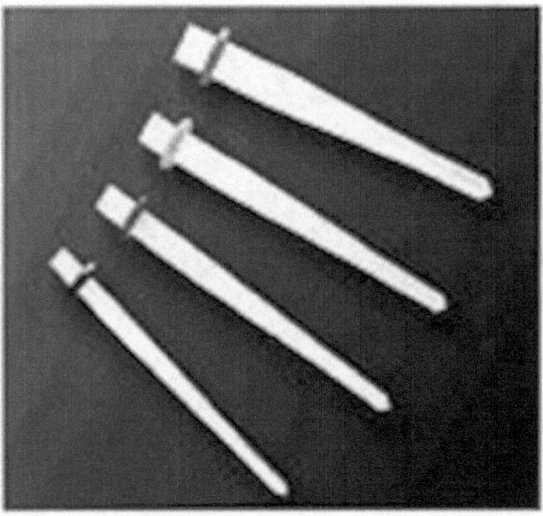

It is a two stage light post. It is made from quartz fibers and it offers comparable mechanical properties, a neutral translucent shade and the added convenience of curing by light energy transmission. With the light post, the bonding primer and the light cure or dual-cure resin cement can be used expediently cured simultaneously in the canal through the post. These posts do not necessitate additional canal preparation as they can easily conform to the root canal anatomy and also they can be placed within the canal and cured. This property helps them to impart strength to the weakened roots thereby reducing the rate of vertical root fracture.

For teeth with large or round roots with substantial amount of root thickness remaining after endodontic treatment is completed, we can choose between either of the post systems. If root thickness required to accommodate a prefabricated post will reduce dentin thickness further then a custom made cast post and core is the safest option.

CORE

The core consists of restorative material placed in the coronal area of the tooth. This material replaces carious, fractured, or otherwise missing coronal structure and retains the final crown. [20]

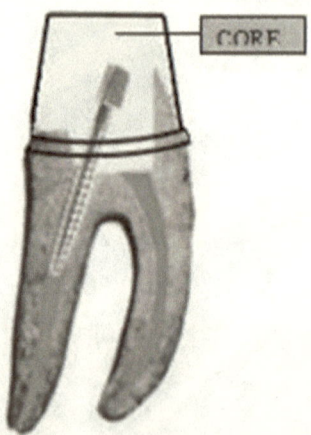

The core is anchored to the tooth by extending into the coronal aspect of the canal or through the endodontic post. The attachment between tooth post and core is mechanical or chemical, as the post and core are usually formed from different materials.

Retention of the core can be augmented by placement of pins, grooves, and channels in the dentin. However these alterations are done at the expense of the remaining tooth structure. Also the use of adhesive resins, the irregular nature of the remaining coronal tooth structure, pulp chamber and canal orifices eliminate the need for such procedures.

Using restorative materials that bond to the tooth structure enhances retention and resistance without the need to remove valuable dentin. Desirable physical properties of core include:-

1. High compressive strength.
2. Dimensional stability.
3. Ease of manipulation.
4. Short setting time.
5. An ability to bond to both the tooth and the post.

Contemporary cores include amalgam, cast metal, composite resin, and glass ionomer cements.

Cast Metal core

A cast metal post and core are a traditional method of restoring endodontically treated teeth. They are indicated in teeth with major coronal destruction. [35]

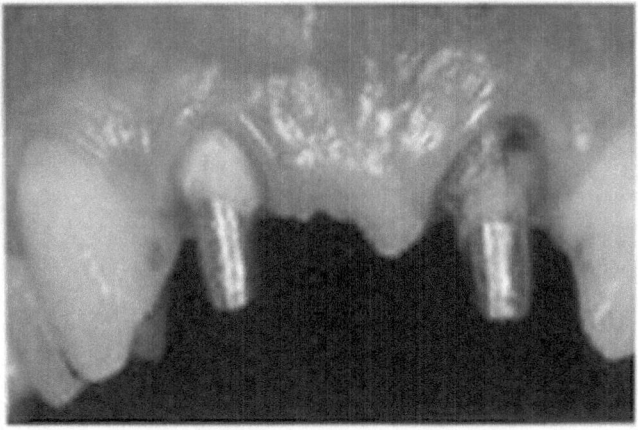

Advantages

1. The core is the integral extension of the post, and the cast core does not depend on the mechanical means for retention on the post.
2. The cast post and core can provide antirotational features with eccentric preparations in the dentin, retentive pins, or a cervical collar at the base of the core. These features also increase the core and crown retention.
3. This construction prevents dislodgement of the core and crown from the post and root when minimal tooth structure remains.
4. Noble metals are non corrosive and ceramo-metal alloys exhibit increased stiffness or decreased dentin deformation.
5. The cast post and core can be used when functional forces on a tooth put the post to core retention at a risk.

Disadvantages

1. The cast post/core system has a higher clinical rate of root fracture than preformed system.
2. Valuable tooth structure is removed to create a path of removal.
3. The procedure is expensive because two appointments are needed and laboratory costs may be significant.
4. The laboratory phase is technique sensitive.
5. Metal casting of a pattern with a large core and a small diameter post can lead to a porosity of the gold at the post-core interface. This results in failure of restoration.
6. Attempts to circumvent this problem by casting a core to a stainless steel preformed post degrade the physical properties of the stainless steel due to the heating and casting procedures in the laboratory.
7. This process results in a foundation restoration:-
    - That is not sufficiently strong to withstand clinical forces.
    - It has corrosive potential.

Amalgam core:

Dental amalgam is a conventional core build up material with a long history of quantifiable success. [35]

- High compressive strength.
- High tensile strength.
- High modulus of elasticity.

These characteristics of amalgam make it an ideal core material.

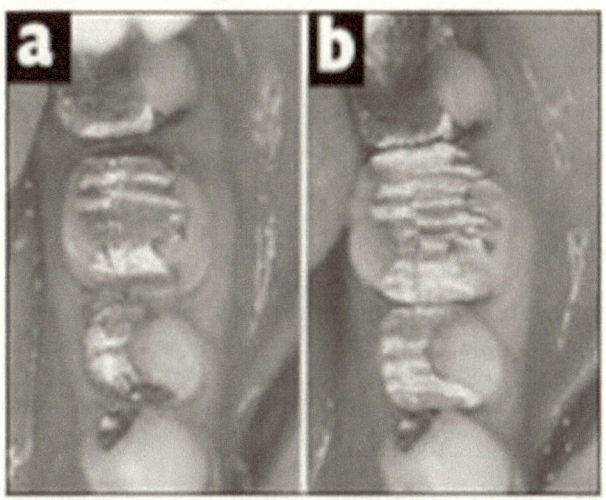

Advantages

1. Amalgam core are highly retentive when used with a preformed post in posterior teeth.
2. Amalgam is easily manipulated and can have a rapid setting time.
3. They require more force to dislodge than cast metal post and cores. This is largely due to high mechanical retention of amalgam to tooth and post undercuts.
4. Supplementary retention and anti rotation can be obtained with auxiliary pins, irregular dentin preparation and dentin bonding agents.

Bonded amalgam demonstrates moderate retention to dentin and has been shown to increase the strength of restored teeth.

5. Amalgam is an economical material. It is easy to use. It is very stable under and functional stresses and therefore transmits minimal stress to the residual tooth structure.
6. When used with dentin bonding agents, the seal at the tooth-alloy junction can be improved by incorporating a layer of resin that chemically bonds to both dentin and metal. The resultant low microleakage discourages recurrent caries and corono-apical endodontic contamination.
7. This core material can be used in almost all teeth where sufficient bulk of amalgam can be easily given and where esthetic is not a primary conscern.

Disadvantages

1. Use of amalgam is declining world wide because of legislative, safety and environmental issues.
2. It cannot be used in teeth in the esthetic zone and also in patients with known allergy to the material.
3. A significant disadvantage is the potential for corrosion and subsequent discoloration of the gingiva or remaining dentin.

Glass ionomer core

Glass ionomer and glass ionomer-silver are adhesive materials useful for small build ups or to fill undercuts in prepared teeth. [35]

It is indicated in teeth in which:-

- ❖ A bulk of core material is possible.
- ❖ Significant sound dentin remains.
- ❖ Moisture control is ensured.
- ❖ Caries control is indicated.

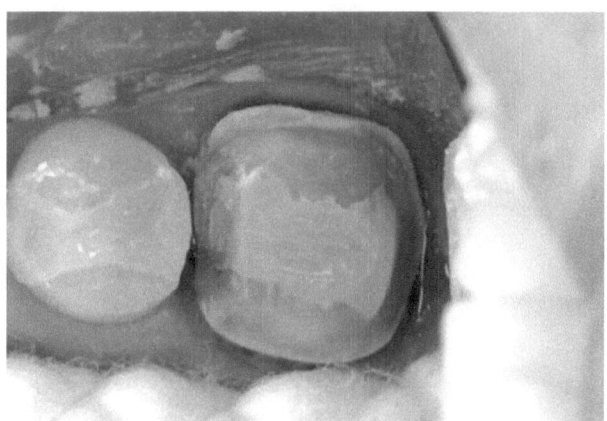

Advantages

1. The major benefit is the anticariogenic property of the material because of the presence of fluoride in the chemical composition.
2. They have low microleakage in comparison to composite resins.
3. They possess adhesive properties.

Disadvantages

1. Glass ionomer is sensitive to moisture as well as soluble in saliva.
2. Glass ionomer cores have low strength and are brittle and are limited to small restorations in which core strength is not required.
3. Low fracture toughness and strength does not favor glass ionomer core in weak anterior teeth or unsupported cusps.
4. Glass ionomer cores demonstrate low retention to preformed metal posts.
5. Adhesive failure can result from contamination of the tooth surface with cutting debris, saliva, blood or protein.

Composite resin core

One of the important core materials is composite resins, which displays favorable ease of manipulation and rapid set. Composite resin has undergone significant development and improvement in its physical characteristics and bond strengths. Preparation for the final restoration is readily accomplished during the core placement session. [35]

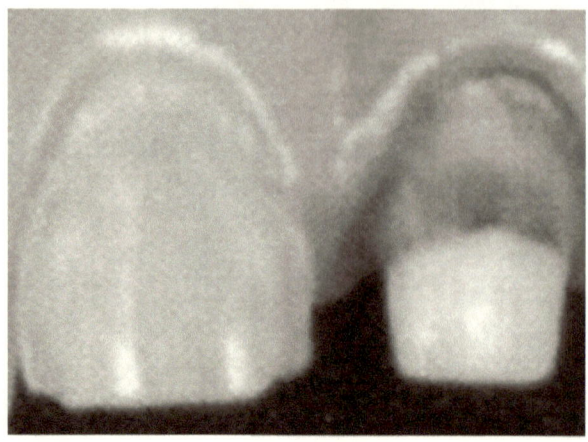

Advantages

1. It bonds adhesively to the tooth structure and resin or zirconia posts.
2. It is easy to manipulate, sets rapidly, translucent or highly opaque formulations, and strong compressive strength. The opaque composite core materials are appropriate for non esthetic areas and enhance visibility during tooth preparation, whereas translucent composite cores enhance esthetics of ceramic restorations.
3. Some formulations which are reinforced with metal or glass fibers can reduce crack propagation through the composite cores.
4. Composite cores have been shown to protect the strength of all ceramic crowns equally as well as stiff amalgam cores. They may provide some protection from root fracture in teeth restored with metal posts compared with amalgam or gold cores.
5. Dentin bonding agents improve the physical characteristics and reduce microleakage of the composite resin core and tooth structure interface, but it requires complete setting of the resin material and it should be compatible with the dentin bonding agents. For example self cure

composite resin requires self cure adhesives; it is incompatible with light cured adhesive.
6. No loss of bond strength occurred when contaminated dentin was cleaned with pumice before bonding of composite core material.
7. The final restoration placement can be readily accomplished during the core placement session itself.

Disadvantages

1. Polymerization shrinkage and contraction away from the tooth structure of non-dentin bonded light cured composite resin can result in microcracks and microleakage at the core-tooth interface.
2. Microleakage exceeds that of amalgam, glass ionomer cement, or glass ionomer resin.
3. It requires a moisture free field for manipulation.
4. No bonding agent completely eliminates microleakage. As a result more than 2 mm of sound tooth structure should remain at the margin for optimal composite resin core function.

Modified glass ionomer core

Resin modified glass ionomer materials are a combination of glass ionomer and composite resin technologies. Therefore they have properties of both the materials. [35]

Advantages

1. They have moderate strength; higher than glass ionomer cement and less than composite resin.
2. It is adequate for moderate sized core build ups.
3. They release fluoride, thereby having an anticariogenic effect.

4. Their bond to dentin is significantly higher than traditional glass ionomer cement and is close to that of dentin bonded composite.
5. Resin modified glass ionomer allows minimal microleakage.

Disadvantages

1. They undergo hygroscopic expansion if they get contaminated with fluid and can cause fracture of ceramic crowns.
2. They have moderate solubility i.e. between that of glass ionomer and composite resins.

CORONAL COVERAGE

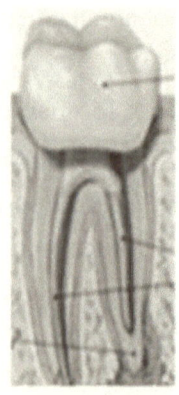

Final Restoration

Pretreatment data review

When it has been determined that post and core is required to properly retain a definitive single crown or a fixed partial denture, following characteristics should be determined prior to beginning the clinical procedures associated with fabrication of a post and core:-

- ❖ Post length.
- ❖ Post diameter.
- ❖ Anatomic or structural limitations.

- Type of post and core that will be used.
- Root selection in multi rooted teeth.
- Type of definitive restoration being placed and its effect on core form and tooth reduction depths.

Post length

Since 5 mm of guttapercha should be retained apically to ensure a good seal, posts should extend to that length in all teeth except molars. With molars posts should be placed in the primary roots and should not be extended more than 7 mm apical to the origin of the root canal in the base of the pulp chamber as extension beyond this can lead to perforations with very little tooth structure remaining.

Post diameter

A frequently used, clinically appropriate guideline for post diameter is not to exceed one-third the root diameter. If it is extended beyond this value, the tooth becomes exponentially weaker. Each millimeter of increase causes a six fold increase in the potential for root fracture.

Studies have determined that post diameter should be about ***0.6 mm for mandibular incisors and 1.0 mm for maxillary central incisors, maxillary and mandibular canines and palatal root of maxillary first molar. For the remaining teeth post diameter was about 0.8 mm.***

Anatomic and structural limitations

After completion of endodontic treatment the tooth should be reviewed before placement of post and core. These characteristics include:-

- The presence and extent of dentine craze lines.
- Identification of teeth for which further root preparation will result in less than 1 mm of remaining dentin or a post diameter greater than one third of the root diameter area.

❖ Information about the areas in which tooth structure is thin.
❖ The point at which significant root curvature begins.

Craze lines

Craze lines in dentine are areas of weakness where further crack propagation may result in root fracture and tooth loss. It is prudent to avoid post placement if possible, in favor of a restorative material core. If a post is required, it should passively fit the canal, and the definitive restoration should entirely encompass the cracked area, whenever possible, by forming a ferrule.

Dentin thickness after endodontic treatment

Following normal and appropriate endodontic instrumentation, teeth can possess less than 1 mm of dentin, indicating that there should be no further root preparation for the post. In such cases it is better to fabricate a post that fits into the existing morphologic form and diameter. This characteristic is one of the primary indications for the use of custom cast post and core. Since mandibular premolars already have an oval or ribbon shaped canal they should not be subjected to any further root preparation for a post as this will result in less than 1 mm of dentin.

Root curvature

When root curvature is present, post length must be limited to preserve remaining dentin, thereby helping to prevent root fracture or perforation. Root curves frequently in the apical 5 mm. Therefore 5mm of guttapercha is retained apically to avoid the curved portions of the roots. Since the roots of molars a frequently curved, the post should terminate at the point where the substantive curvature begins.

Type of post and core

Posts can be Classified as cemented or threaded.

Cemented posts depend on their proximity to prepared dentin walls and cementing medium. Whereas threaded posts depend primarily on engaging the tooth – either through the threads formed in the dentin as the post is screwed into the root or through threads previously 'tapped' into the dentin.

Type of definitive restoration

It is important to know the type of single crown or retainer i.e. all metal, all ceramic, metal ceramic that will be used as a final restoration. This helps us to plan the amount of tooth reduction in accordance with that required for each type of restoration.

TECHNIQUES FOR RESTORATION OF ENDODONTICALLY TREATED TEETH RESTORATIONS WITHOUT POSTS

- ❖ Posterior teeth with small restorations, sufficient remaining tooth structure, or both, should be restored with cast restorations covering the occlusal surface, e.g. onlay, partial veneer crowns. A heavy reverse bevel is recommended over the cusps for further protection. [27]
- ❖ For patients with reduced tooth structure, a complete crown is indicated. If core is needed, it is placed using the coronal pulp chamber for retention.

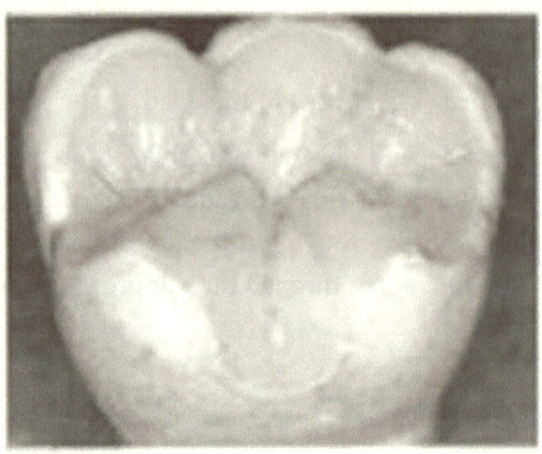

RESTORATIONS WITH POSTS

❖ Two types of posts are used in endodontically treated teeth; the prefabricated and the custom cast post and cores. Prefabricated posts are more appropriately used for multi rooted teeth to support an amalgam or in some cases a composite core buildup. Whereas custom cast post and core is indicated for most single rooted teeth.

PROCEDURE

The principles of preparation for a post and core are that:-

1. All useful tooth structure should be preserved.
2. The apical seal is maintained.
3. Stress in minimized within the tooth and post and core.

Tooth preparation for endodontically treated teeth can be considered as a multi-staged operation:- [19]

1. Establishing the post length.
2. Removal of the root canal filling material to appropriate depth.
3. Enlargement and shaping of canal
4. Develop antirotation features.

5. Preparation of coronal tooth structure.
6. Finishing procedures.

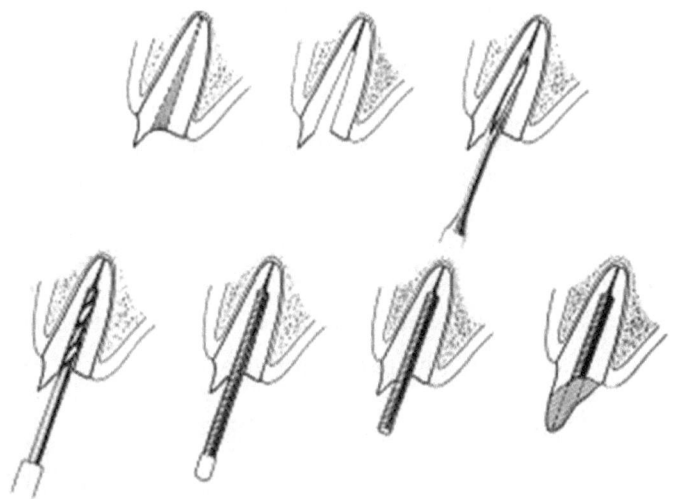

1. ***Establishing post length***

    This should be carried out once the temporary restoration has been removed from the tooth. At this stage the coronal landmarks remain, that will have previously provided reference for root canal treatment. The length can only be determined from reference to a good quality radiograph.

    From which we can also determine:-

    ❖ The overall shape of the root, particularly the width in the apical third.
    ❖ The apparent width of the root canal.
    ❖ The length of the clinical crown.
    ❖ The level of alveolar bone surrounding the root.
    ❖ The approximate length of the root itself.

    The shape of the root and the width of the canal will determine whether the post can be parallel sided or threaded or tapered. The post should occupy no more than one third of the radiographic width of the root at the apical end of the post.

2. ***Removal of the root canal filling to appropriate depth***

   A root canal filling of guttapercha can be removed either immediately following root canal filling or at the time of preparation for the post. Guttapercha can be removed by heating a root canal plugger and placing it in the canal to begin the preparation for the post. On removal portions of the softened filling with adhere to the instrument. This is repeated until the desired penetration is reached. System B can also be used to remove guttapercha. It has a plugger with a rubber plug to maintain the length of guttapercha removal. [8]

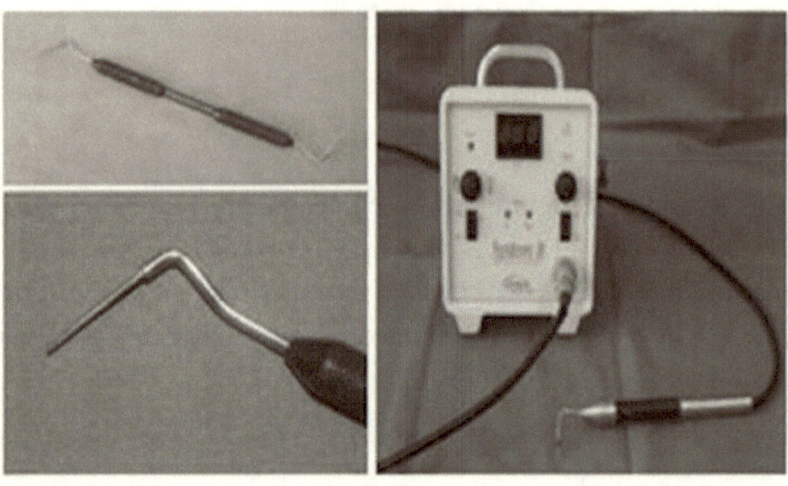

Rotary instruments can also be used like Gates Glidden burs and Peeso reamers [the initial diameter of the GGD should be less than the diameter of the root canal]. They are used when the guttapercha has lost its thermo plasticity and is old; making sure that the instrument follows the guttapercha and does not cut into the dentin. Rotary instruments are faster but have a potential to cause root perforation if done improperly. Care should be taken to preserve the guttapercha in the apical 5 mm of the root. Solvents should be avoided as they can disturb the apical seal. [19]

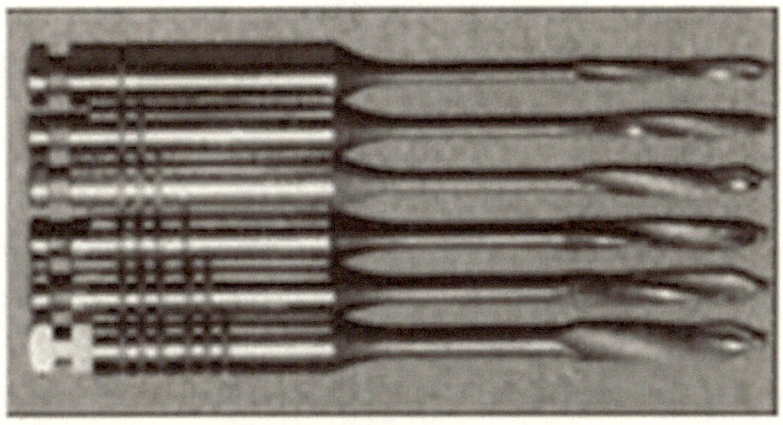

3. ***Enlargement and shaping of the canal***

   ❖ When guttapercha has been removed to appropriate depth, shape the canal as needed. This is done using endodontic hand instruments or a low speed twist drills and hand reamers used serially to widen the canal so that post will contact solid dentin rather than canal filling material.

   ❖ If the canal is sclerotic and enlargement becomes tedious the use of canal irrigants or chelating agents becomes helpful. Non-end cutting instruments such as Gates Glidden drills can be used carefully to widen the canal in preparation for reamers, twist drills, 10:1 gear reduction hand pieces with light pressure without forcing and depth stops. [19]

   ❖ The purpose is to remove undercuts and prepare the canal to receive appropriately sized post without excessively enlarging the canal. Prior to enlargement of the canal the type of post system should be decided.

   ❖ In case of a prefabricated threaded post, the appropriate drill is followed by a tap. Parallel sided posts are more retentive and distribute stresses better than tapered posts, but they do not conform to the shape of the canal that has been flared to facilitate condensation of guttapercha. Then a tapered custom made post is preferred. A tapered post will conform better to the canal than a parallel sided post and will need less removal of dentin to achieve an adequate fit. However it will be less retentive and will cause greater stress concentrations.

- ❖ Parallel sided prefabricated posts are recommended for conservatively prepared root canals in teeth with roots of circular cross section. Excessively flared canals may be found in young patients, or following retreatment of an endodontic failure, are best managed with a custom post.
- ❖ We should be careful not to remove more dentin than necessary the apical end.

4. **Anti rotation features**

    - ❖ The form of post preparation is essential if dentine is to be preserved and stresses are to be minimized.
    - ❖ A tapered post will reflect the essential anatomy of the root canal. It will be widened coronally in order to increase the bulk of the post especially where the post joins the core. This widening is carried out bucco-lingually in the coronal half of the root. It should not be overemphasized to avoid unnecessary dentin loss. It is done using Gates Glidden drill as it will not produce sharp angles and thus will minimize stress concentration.
    - ❖ When the post is parallel sided, it should be tapered in its coronal portion, reflecting the normal anatomy of the root canal. Rapid changes in the bulk of the material and consequently sharp line angles will promote stress concentration and will increase the possibility of fracture.
    - ❖ The apical portion of the post preparation should be completed before the coronal preparation. The final apical preparation is carried out with a parallel sided twist drill which cuts on its tip; therefore it should be used by hand to minimize the chances of

perforation. These drills should be withdrawn from the canal at frequent intervals and the canal should be cleaned of debris. [19]

- ❖ The coronal part of the root canal is then prepared and blended into the radicular portion, such that sharp changes in direction are avoided and stress minimized.
- ❖ There is no need for notching of the root canal or root face both of which will be detrimental in terms of stress concentration.

5. *Preparation of coronal tooth structure*

After the post space has been prepared, the coronal tooth structure is reduced for extra coronal restoration. The amount of tooth structure that needs to be removed is related to the type of crown to be used, and that, in turn determines the extent of core fabrication. For instance if some of the remaining tooth structure is very thin after the coronal preparation, it is better to remove that part of dentin and replace it as a part of core.

POST AND CORE FABRICATION

Prefabricated cemented or bonded post/restorative material core[19]

1. Root canal filling material is removed until the desired post depth is achieved.
2. The canal is enlarged in size, so that the selected post should fit passively into the prepared canal without any substantial movement. At least the apical half of the post should fit closely to the preparation. The coronal half may not fit due to canal flaring, which will be corrected when the post is fabricated around it.

3. Care must be taken not to remove more dentin than necessary at the apical end.

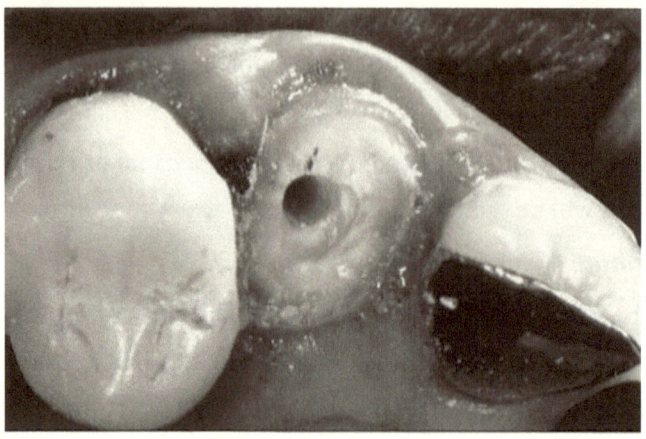

4. Radiographic conformation is essential to ensure proper seating and length of post.

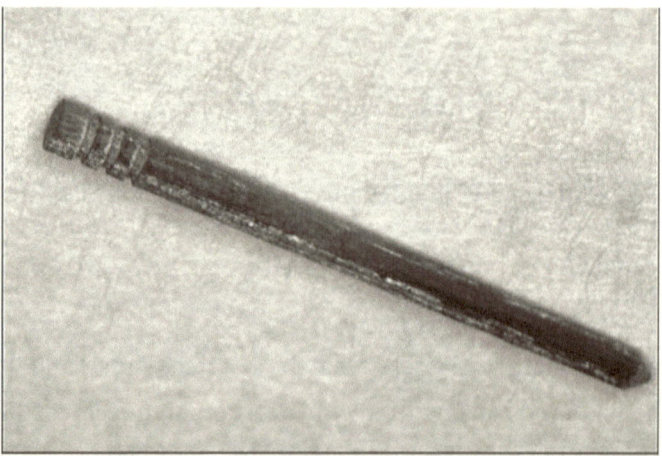

5. The incisal or occlusal end of the post is shortened so that is done not interfere with the opposing occlusion, but it must provide support and retention for the restorative core material.

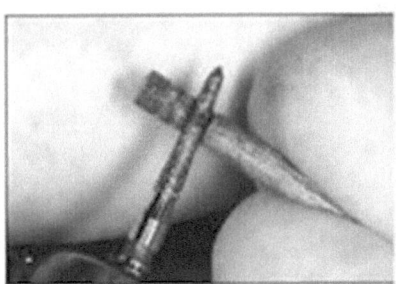
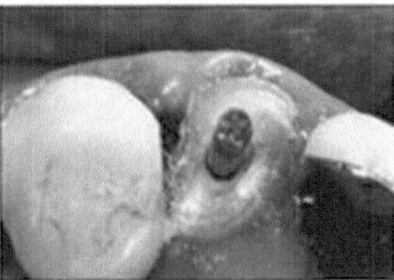

6. When metal posts are used they can be bent coronally to align them within the core material. Post bending is done outside the mouth.

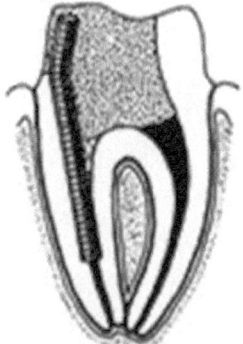
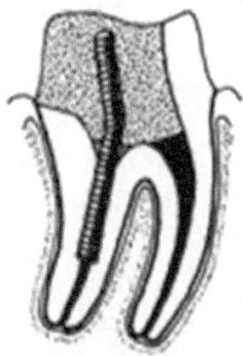

7. The post is cemented into the root canal using resin bonding procedures.

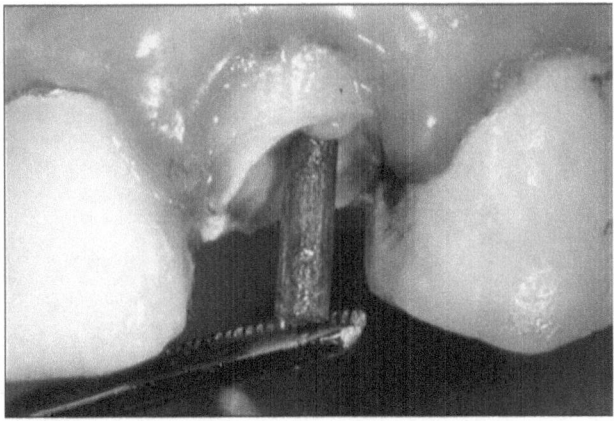

8. Restorative material is then condensed around the post or bonded to the post and remaining tooth structure. A slight excess of material is placed, and this is removed during crown preparation.

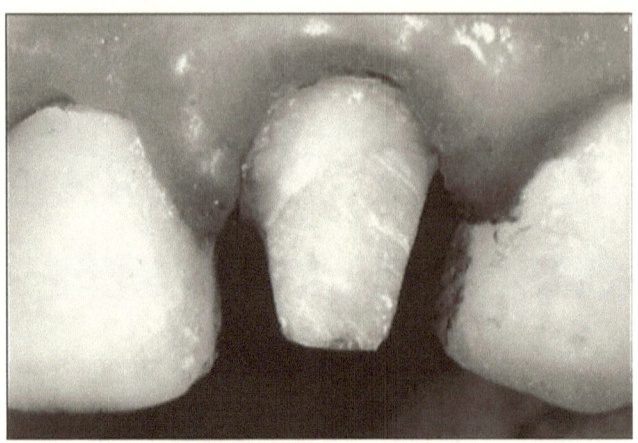

9. The definitive tooth preparation is then completed and impression is made for the crown.

Prefabricated threaded post / restorative material core

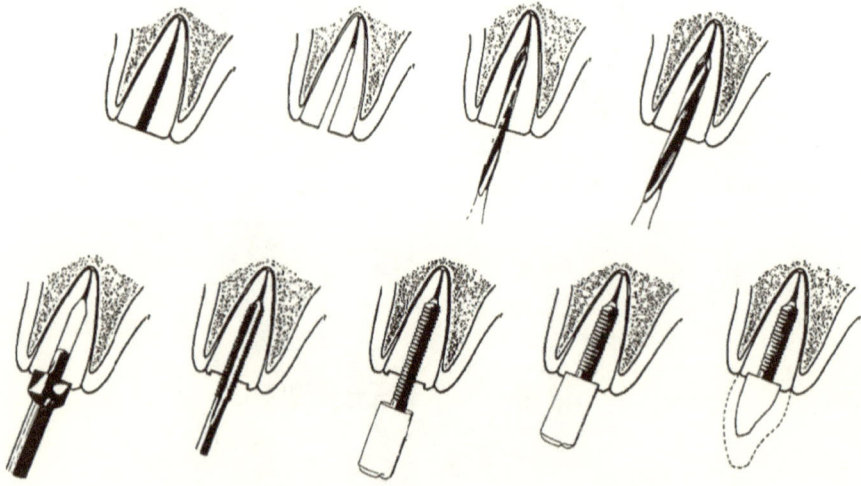

1. The root canal filling material is removed as described.
2. The canal is sequentially enlarged using manufacturers instructions until the desired diameter is achieved. This also determines the size of the tap and the post that will be used.
3. The Kurer post system uses a root facer system to prepare a flat area on the coronal surface of the root (countersink) against which the incorporated core is seated.
4. Then the root is threaded using hand taps or post is threaded into the canal
5. Trial placement of the post is done to verify how much of the post must be shortened.
6. After the post is in place, the core is formed by reshaping the attached metal core to form a shape that represents the shape of a prepared tooth and will provide appropriate space for fabrication of a crown. [19]

Custom - Cast Post and Core

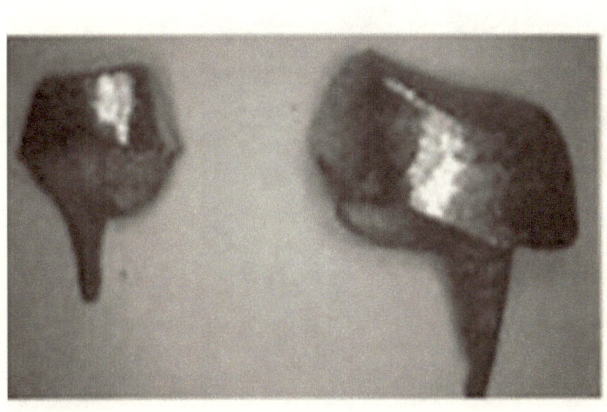
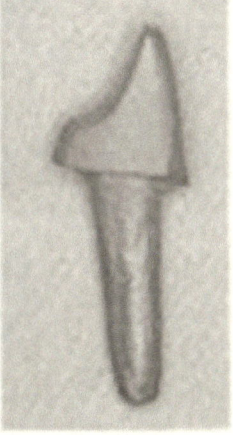

- ❖ Using either direct or indirect techniques, cast post and core can be fabricated for the treated tooth.
- ❖ The root canal filling material is removed as described earlier. It is not desirable to make the post space round.

- Since most custom-cast post and cores possess a slightly tapered form, a flat area should be prepared on the coronal tooth structure perpendicular to the long axis of the post which serves as a positive stop during cementation of the post and during application of thereby helping to minimize any tendency for the post to wedge against the tooth.

Direct technique

In direct technique a castable post and core pattern is fabricated directly on the prepared tooth in the patients' mouth.

Steps

1. Select a plastic post that fits within the confines of the post preparation without binding. Leave the post sufficiently long so that it can be grasped for easy placement and removal.

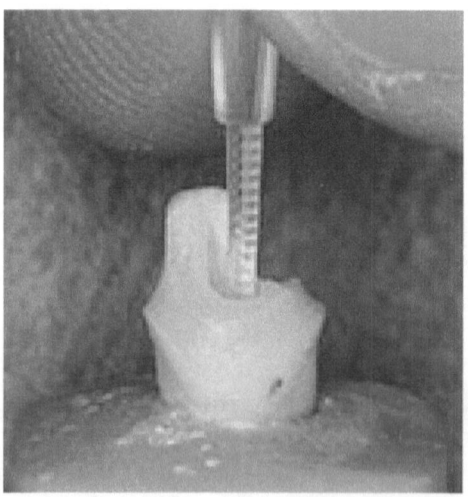

2. Lightly lubricate the canal using a water soluble lubricant such as die lubricant helps ensure that all lubricant can be consequently removed, thereby not interfering with cement retention.

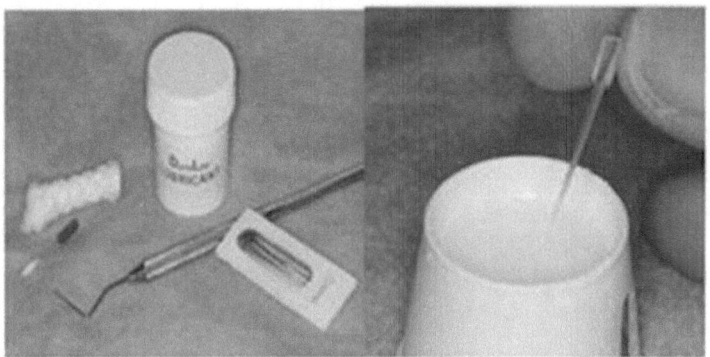

3. Place notches on the side of the plastic post pattern if the post is smooth and place it to the depth of the prepared canal.
4. Use the bead brush technique to apply resin to the prepared canal and the body of the post and seat the post in the canal.

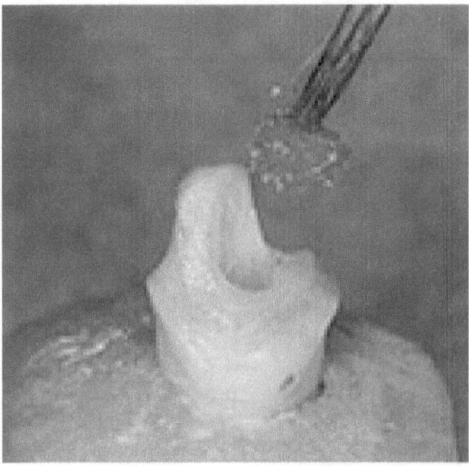

5. Do not allow the resin to completely harden within the canal. Remove and reseat the post and attached resin several times while the resin is still in its rubbery stage so that the pattern does not inadvertently become locked into the canal.

6. Remove the polymerized pattern and inspect the resin for lack of voids. Reseat the post and test for adaptation and passivity.

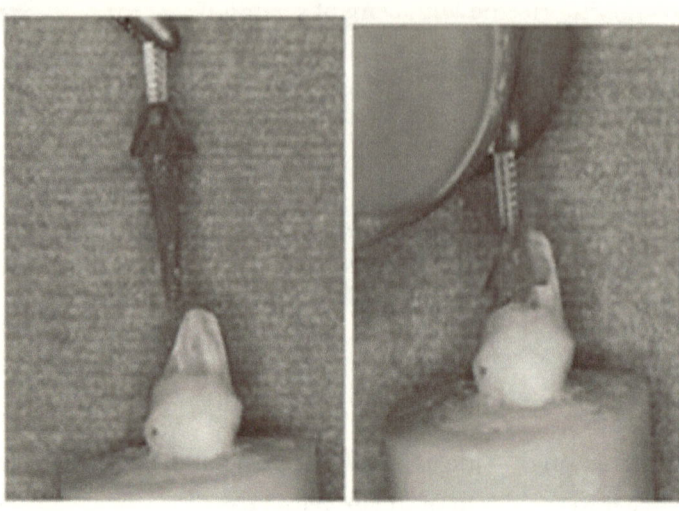

7. Add additional coronal resin to form the desired dimensions of the core. Remove and reseat the pattern as described previously to prevent it from becoming locked into the coronal tooth structure. A slight excess of core resin is added so that the hardened core can be prepared with a high speed diamond bur and water spray to the desired form

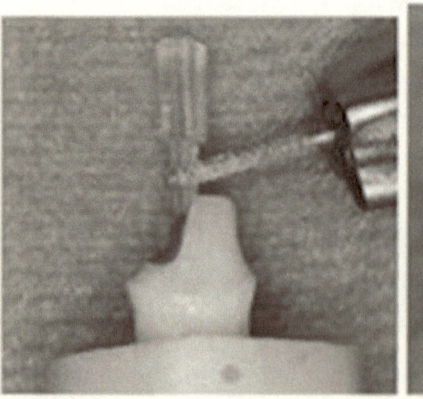
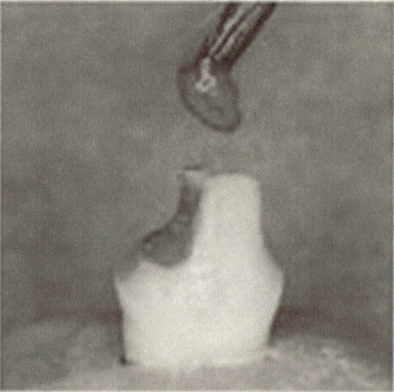

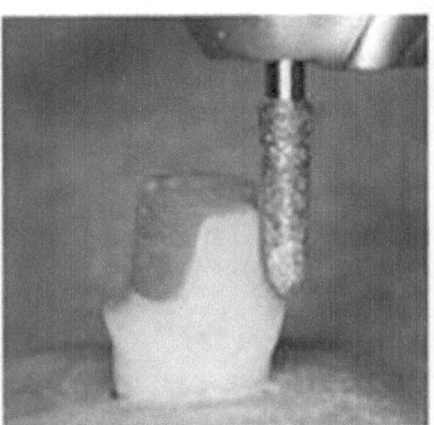 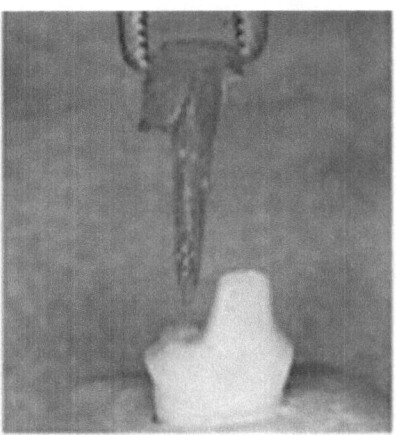

8. The core is then removed, invested, and cast.

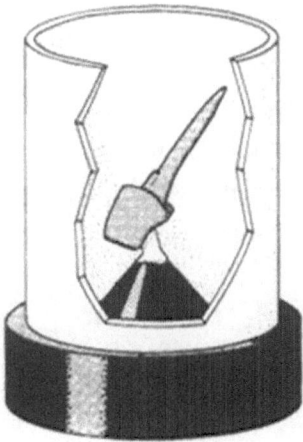

9. A temporary crown is given to the patient in the mean time. This is known as **temporization**. [19] A temporary restoration must do the following:-
   * Seal coronally, preventing ingress of coronal fluids and bacteria and egress of intracanal medicaments.
   * Enhance isolation during treatment procedures.
   * Protect tooth structure until final restoration is placed.

10. The post and the core are trial placed, adjusted and then cemented. Then the definitive tooth preparation can be completed.
11. A pattern can also be prepared using wax rather than resin.

Indirect technique

The indirect technique uses an impression and stone dye of the tooth for the pattern fabrication.

Steps

1. Non aqueous elastomeric impression materials make accurate impressions of the prepared root canal, but some method of supporting the impression material prevents distortion/displacement of the set material during removal from the mouth and pouring of the cast.
2. Several methods of support are available. A metal wire that returns to its original shape when slightly distorted is desirable. Safety pins and orthodontic wires have been used for this purpose. [19]

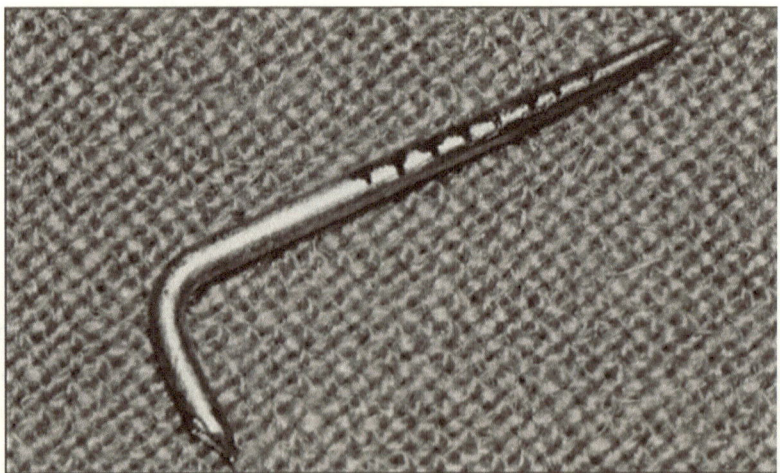

3. Metal wire such as a paper clip can be bent on impression removal and can be permanently distorted. Plastic posts are also used to support the impression material. They can be flexed in slightly curved canal or if they contact coronal tooth structure. Subsequent removal of the post

after the impression material sets allows straightening of the plastic post to occur, which results in distortion.

4. Only use plastic posts when they are totally passive and do not bind on any tooth structure.
5. When a safety pin or orthodontic wire is selected as the means of supporting the impression material, the coronal portion of the wire should be bent over to form a handle and to help retain it in the impression material.
6. Notch the wire and coat it with adhesive.
7. Fill the prepared canal with impression material using a slowly rotating lentulospiral instrument (DENTSPLY Maillefer) accompanied by an up and down motion. [8, 19]

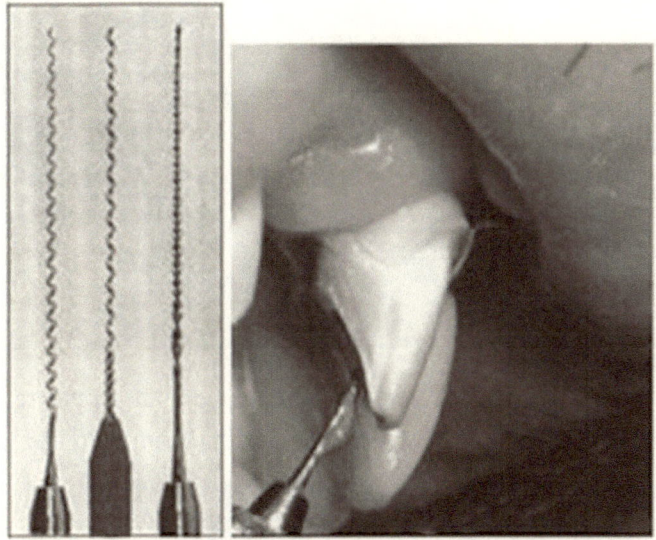

8. Alternately, an anesthetic needle can be placed to the depth of the post space (to serve as an air escape channel) and impression material syringed down the canal.
9. Seat the wire or plastic post through the impression material to the full depth of the canal, syringe additional impression material around the supporting device as well as the prepared tooth, and seat the impression tray.

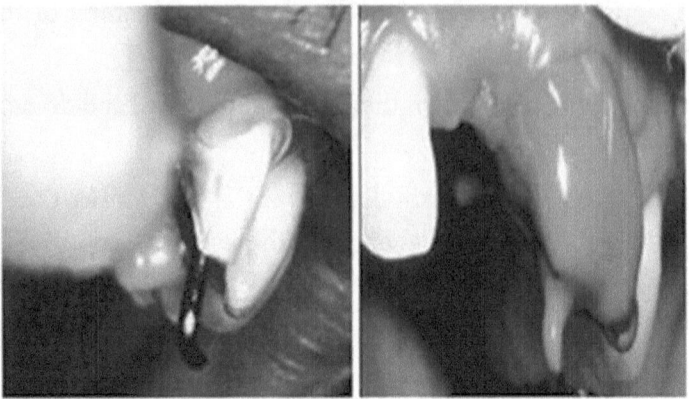

10. Remove the impression, evaluate it and pour a cast.

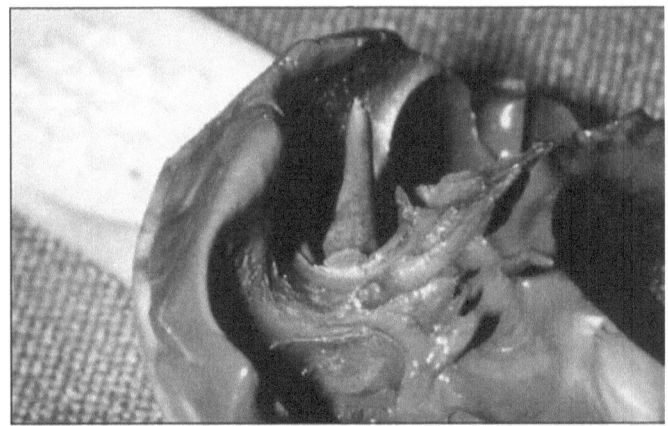

11. Make an interocclusal record and obtain an opposite cast and appropriately sized plastic post to be used in forming a wax pattern.

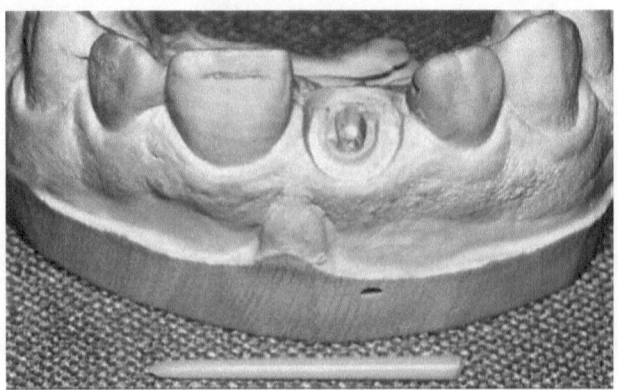

12. Lightly lubricate the canal of the working cast with die lubricant.

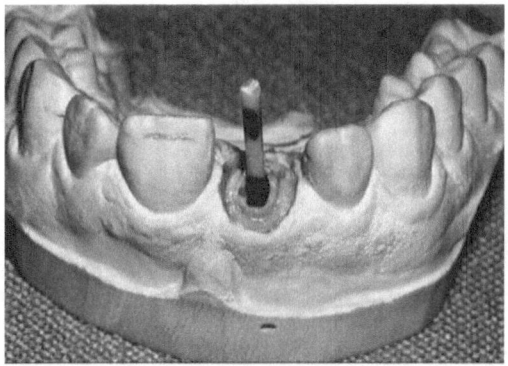

13. Place notches on the side of the plastic post and then add soft inlay wax in small increments, fully seating the plastic post after each increment of wax is added.

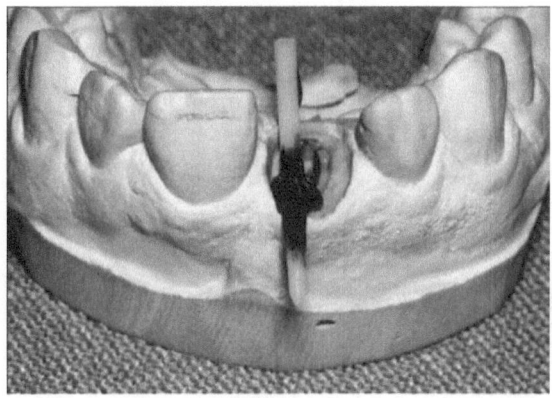

14. Ensure that the pattern is well adapted but passive.

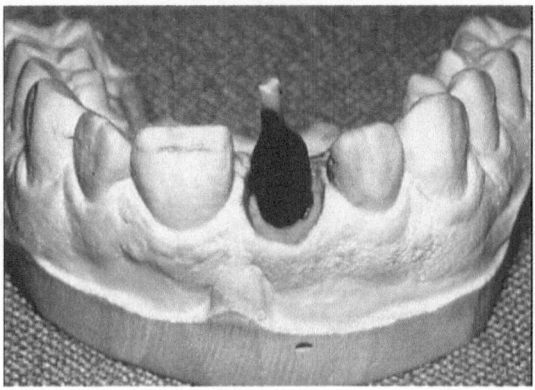

15. After the post pattern has been fabricated, the wax core is added and shaped, and then the pattern is cast in metal.

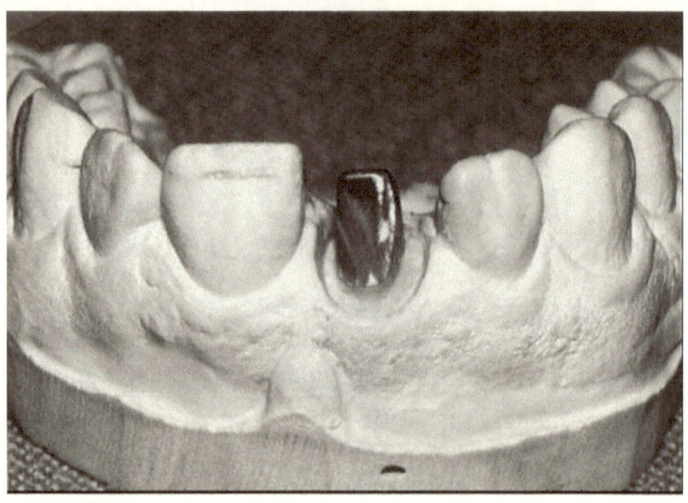

16. The cast post and core are then cemented in the tooth and definitive tooth preparation is completed.

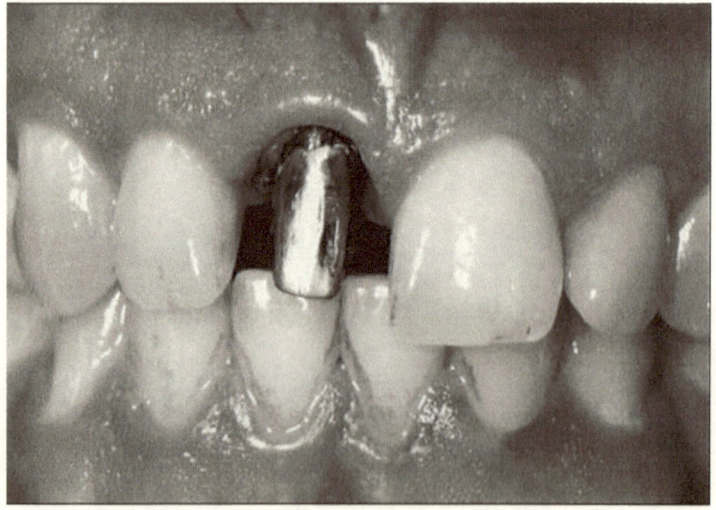

CAST POSTS AND CORES FOR MULTIROOTED TEETH

On occasions there may be such a lack of coronal dentin in a posterior tooth that demands placed on a plastic core material becomes unrealistic.

Dentists understandably like to have a *'rule of thumb'* for when this point is reached. However, it is not possible to be entirely perspective as the decision depends on:

1. The quantity or remaining tooth structure.
2. The quality of dentin.
3. The load that will act on the tooth and restoration.

Number of posts

The availability of more than one root canal has traditionally often meant that more than one post can be placed. In terms of loss of dentin, such an approach is not always valid. Additional posts may help to distribute stresses to those roots in which they are placed, but this needs to be balanced against the knowledge that posts do not produce reinforcement.

Antirotation

Resistance to rotation is generally more easily achieved in multi rooted teeth due to the availability of a definitive pulp chamber. When it needs to be enhanced internally it should be done where maximum dentin is present.

Indications for multiple posts

1. When the root selected for the post is short or when the anatomy of the root prevents it being used till the desired length.
2. When there is little in the way of the pulp chamber to provide antirotation.

Direct pattern

A direct pattern can be used for multi rooted teeth. A single piece core with auxiliary posts is used as opposed to the multisection core recommended for indirect posterior cast post and cores. The core is cast directly onto the post of one canal. The other canals already have prefabricated posts that pass through holes in the core. [32]

Steps

1. Smooth parallel sided or tapered posts are used.

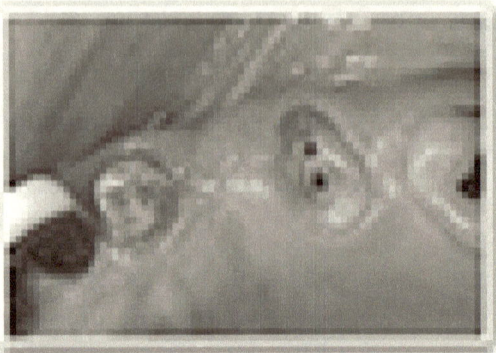

2. Fit prefabricated posts into the prepared canal. One post is roughened; the others are left smooth and lubricated. All posts should extend beyond the eventual preparation.

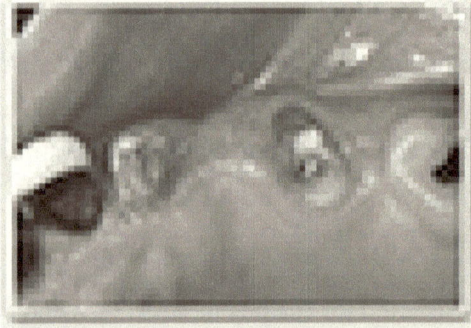

3. Build up the core by autopolymerising resin by the bead technique.

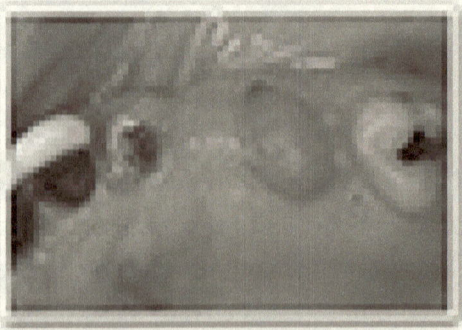

4. Shape the core to final form with carbide finishing burs.

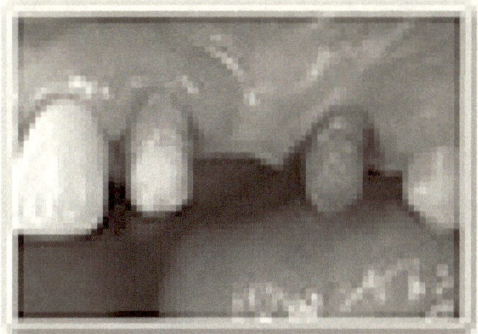

5. Grip the smooth lubricated posts with forceps and remove them.
6. Remove, invest and cast the core with the roughened post.
7. When this has been done, the holes for the auxiliary posts can be refined with the appropriate twist drill.

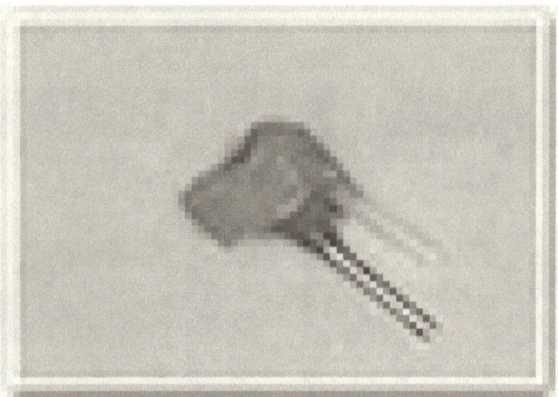

8. After verifying the fit at try-in, cement the core and auxiliary posts to place. [32]

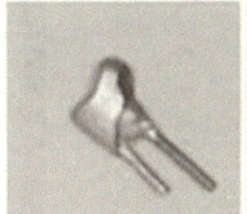 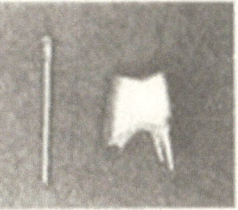 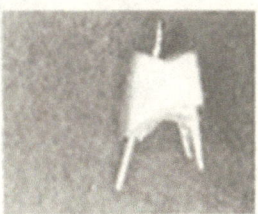

Indirect pattern

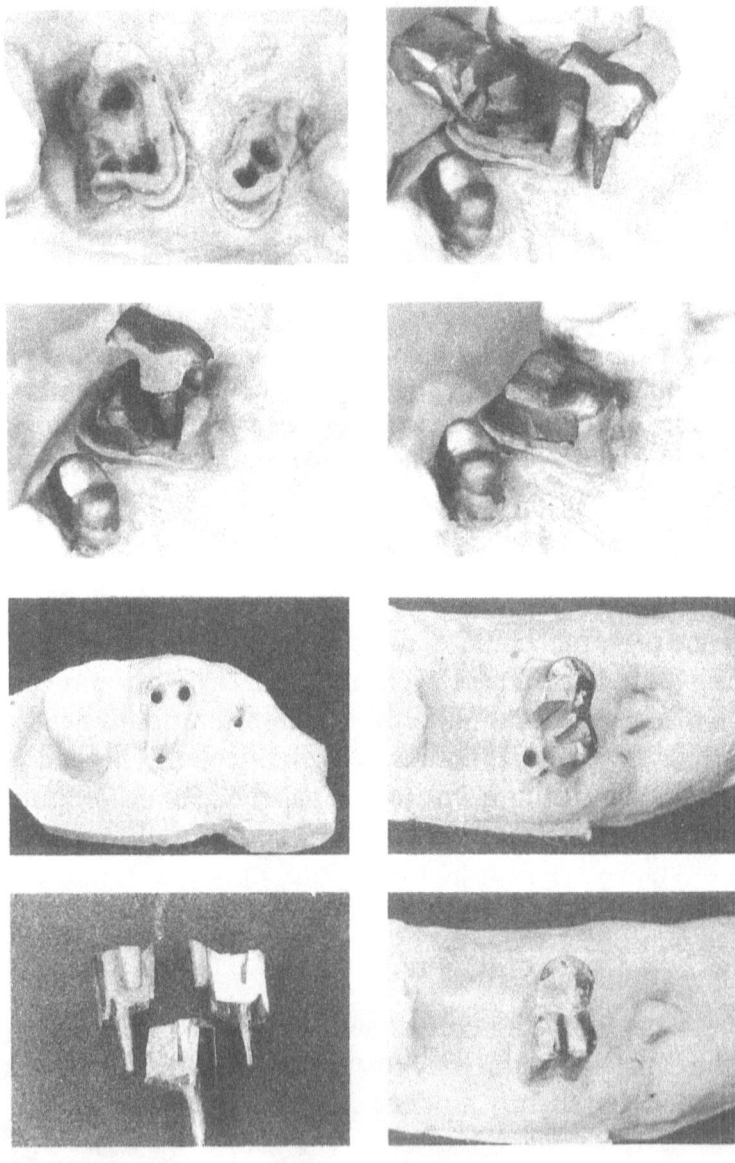

Steps

1. Wax the custom made posts as described earlier.
2. Build part of the core around the first post.
3. Remove any undercuts adjacent to other post holes and cast the first section.
4. Wax additional sections and cast them.
5. The use of dovetails to interlock the sections makes the procedure more complicated and is probably of limited benefit, especially because the final buildup is held together by the fixed cast restoration. [32]

REMOVAL OF EXISTING POSTS

Occasionally, an existing post and core must be removed e.g. for retreatment of a failed root canal filling. If sufficient length of post is exposed coronally, the post can be retrieved with thin beaked forceps. Vibrating the post first with an ultrasonic scaler will weaken the cement and facilitate its removal. A thin scaler tip is also recommended. Alternatively, a post puller can be used. This device consists of a vise to grip the post and legs that bear on the root face. A screw activates the vise and extracts the post. [8]

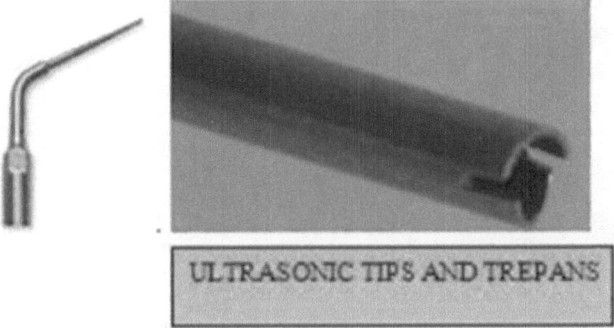

ULTRASONIC TIPS AND TREPANS

A post that has fractured within the root canal cannot be removed with a post puller or forceps. The post can be drilled out, but great care is needed to avoid deviation. This technique is best limited to relatively short fractured posts.[8]

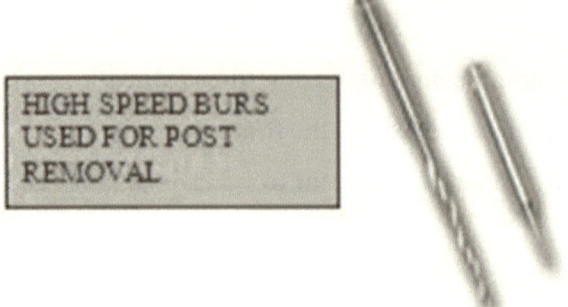

HIGH SPEED BURS USED FOR POST REMOVAL

Another means of handling an embedded fractured post (described by *Massernan* in 1966) uses special hollow end cutting tubes (or **trephines**) to prepare a thin trench around the post. The technique has proved to be quite successful. Retrieval can be facilitated by using an adhesive to attach a hollow tube extractor or by using a threaded extractor. [8, 19]

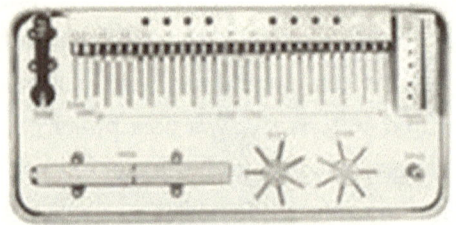

MASSERANS' POST REMOVAL KIT.

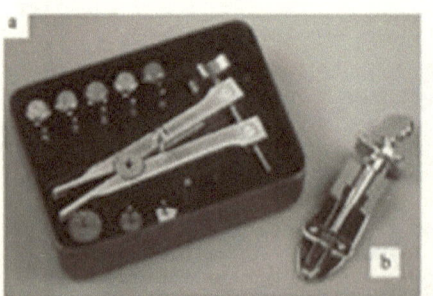

RUDDLE AND EGGLER SYSTEMS FOR POST REMOVAL.

FINAL TOOTH COVERAGE

It can be done by various means:-

Laminates

Laminates are veneer like restorations. They restore the facial surface of the tooth for esthetic purposes. They are made up of either composite resins or porcelains. Laminate bonding is indicated for a combination of mild to moderate anomalies of color, position and form of teeth. As endodontically treated teeth usually become dull and darker in shade, restoring them with laminates helps in improving esthetics.

They are used when sufficient tooth structure remains and there the main concern is for esthetics. [28]

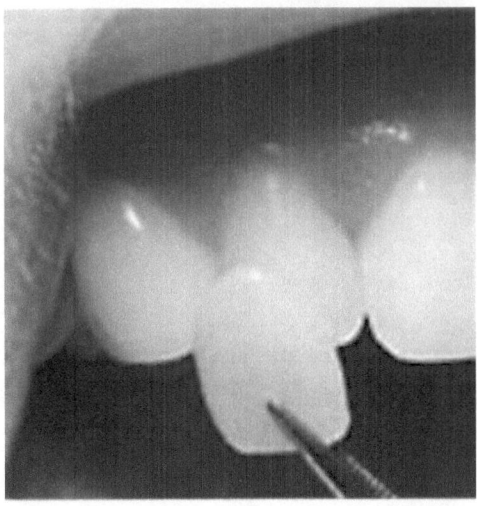

Partial jacket crowns

Partial jacket crowns are restorations covering two or more surfaces of a tooth. The rationale is to enhance the esthetics of the restoration and to conserve the tooth structure. Used mostly for anterior teeth.

- ❖ *Indicated:* in intact teeth with average crown length and normal anatomic form. Loss of part or whole of the tip of the tooth through trauma.
- ❖ *Contraindicated:* in short teeth or teeth with extensive crown restoration.

Advantage: they require less tooth reduction.

Types of partial jacket crowns

a. **Three-quarter crown:-** They restore the occlusal surface and three of the four axial surfaces not including the facial surface. [29]

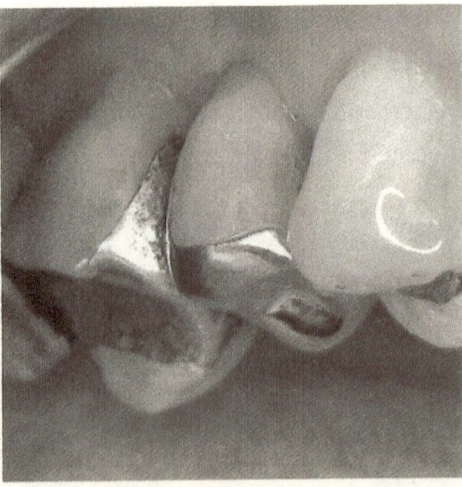

b. **Reverse three-quarter crown:-** They restore all the surfaces except the lingual surface. They are usually indicated in mandibular molars with severe lingual inclination.

c. **Seven-eighth crown:-** They are extensions of three quarter crowns to include major portion of the facial surface. They are generally indicated for maxillary molars and premolars where mesial surface of the tooth is sound, but the distal surface has been destroyed by caries. [29]

Full crowns

They restore and cover all the surfaces of the crown. They are used mostly in posterior teeth.

Types of full crowns

a. **Full metal crown:-** They are made up of cast metal alloys and are usually indicated in areas where there are heavy occlusal loads and esthetics is not of much importance.

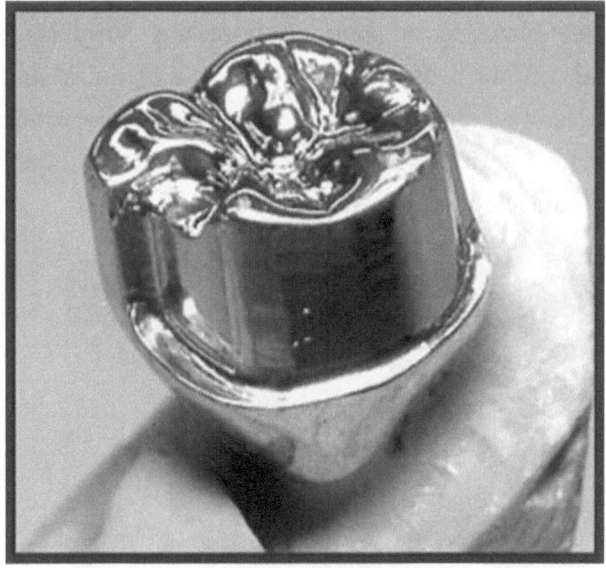

b. **Porcelain fused to metal crown:-** These crowns consist of a cast metal substructure, to which porcelain is fused. Usually gold is used as a substructure, but these days use of base metal alloys is increasing. The remaining tooth structure needs to be reduced nearly 2 mm on the facial surface to allow for the bulk of the porcelain, and 1 to 1.5 mm on the rest of the surfaces. In the cervical area, it is often difficult to mask the metal and in some cases it is left exposed, especially in the posterior areas. [27, 29]

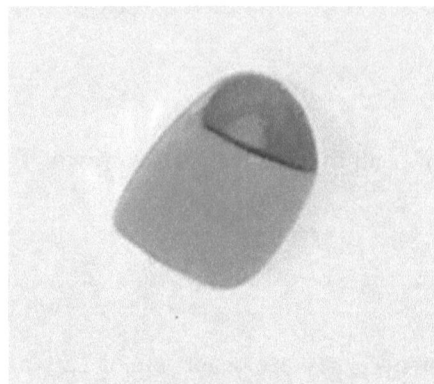

c. **Feldspathic porcelain jacket crown:-** These are translucent porcelain crowns which can be altered to match natural teeth in shade by appropriate blending of standard porcelain powders. The desired shape and contour is usually fabricated on a platinum matrix that has been adapted to a die representing the abutment preparation. They are indicated for anterior teeth, they have superior esthetic quality, but they are easily subjected to fracture. [27, 29]

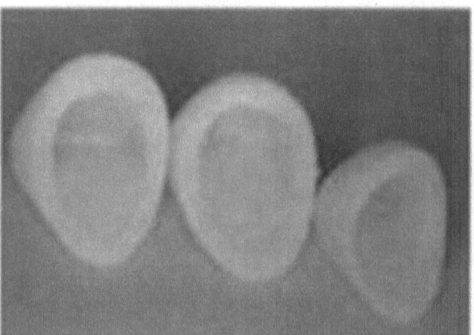

d. **Aluminous porcelain jacket crown:-** The core of this crown is composed of approximately 50% dental porcelain. Such type of core increases the strength of restoration. Since alumina is an opaque material, this type of jacket crown does not have a translucency exhibited by the feldspathic crown.

e. **Bonded alumina crown:-** In this crown, the aluminous porcelain is bonded to pure platinum foil. The purpose of this is to improve strength by eliminating the micro cracks present on the inner surface of the ceramic. The lining of porcelain remains a part of the crown.

f. **Cerestore crown:-** This crown is a ceramic restoration that uses a shrink free alumina ceramic core with an aluminous porcelain veneer. The high strength alumina core makes this crown best suited for restoration of posterior teeth. It offers superior esthetics. The only disadvantage being complex technique for fabrication. [27,29]

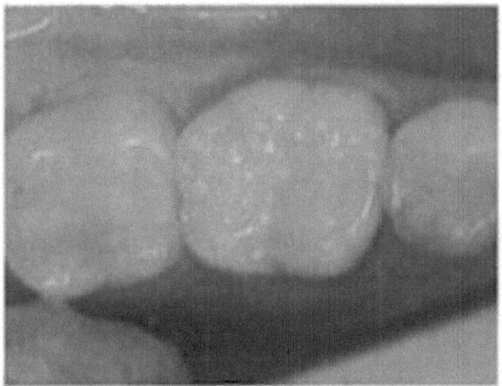

g. **Dicor crown:-** This crown is truly castable ceramic restoration that has sufficient strength for use in posterior teeth. It is translucent and offers superior esthetics. The advantage is that occlusion and anatomy can be predetermined in wax pattern on an articulated cast. [27]

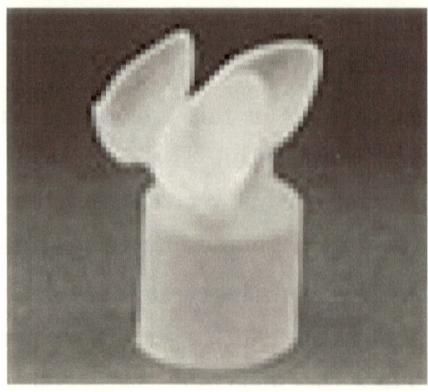

FAILURE OF POST AND CORE RESTORATIONS

Clinical evaluation of crowned teeth with posts reported that 10% of all the failures were due to root fracture. *5% is due to loosening of posts. 2%—4% of the roots fracture and the incidence of apical problems and caries are higher in teeth with posts.* [20]

Failure can occur at many levels

1. **At the apical end:**- Due to removal of excess guttapercha from the apical end of the root. This can lead to secondary caries and apical pathosis due to microleakage from microenvironment.
2. **Loosening of the post from the root canal:**- This can occur due to decementation of the posts which are cemented into the canal, or also due to the dissolution of the cement used.
3. **Fracture of posts can occur:**- Resiliency of the posts is its ability to deflect elastically under force without permanent damage; it is a valuable quality in the post. Posts made of non stiff material are more resilient, absorb more impact force, and transmit less force to the root rather than stiff posts. When they are subjected to higher forces they may fracture.

4. **Root fracture:-** In a clinical study conducted of vertical root fractures, 91% of the teeth had poorly designed posts described as "too long or too wide or both". Posts that are too short also create damaging stresses in the root contributing to root fracture. Posts are made from stiff materials (having high modulus of elasticity) are resistant to flexion under force. Teeth with minimal tooth structure must rely on the post to hold the crown in place. Since rigid posts bend and flex less than non rigid posts, they can limit the movement of the core and possible disruption of the crown margins and cement seal. However, the force must go somewhere, so the force from a stiff post is transmitted to the root, next to the apex of the post. Tapered posts produce a wedging effect on the roots causing them to fracture more than parallel sided posts.

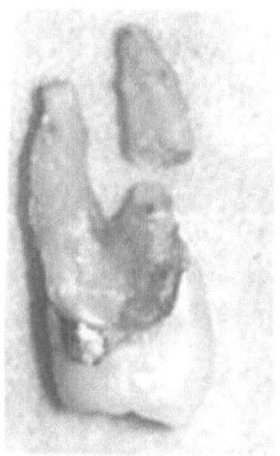

5. Since the most important part of the restored tooth is the tooth itself, it cannot be substituted for by any other material. If there is no sufficient tooth structure remaining chances are that it would lead to failure of restoration because there is nothing to support the restoration being placed in the tooth.

OVERDENTURES

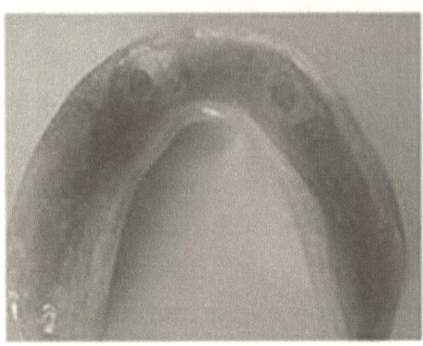 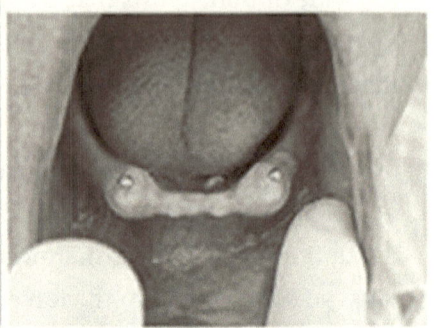

An **overdenture** is a complete denture supported by retained teeth and the residual alveolar ridge. Because the retained teeth are shortened, contoured, and altered to be covered, they need to be treated endodontically.

In 1969, **Lord and Teel** coined the term *'overdenture'* and described the combined endodontic-periodontic-prosthodontic technique applied thereto.

As early as 1916, however, **Prothero** had referred to the use of root support, stating, "*Often two or three widely separated roots or teeth can be utilized for supporting a denture*". It should also be noted that much earlier, in 1789, George Washington's first lower denture, constructed of ivory by **John Greenwood**, was in part supported by a left mandibular premolar. Retaining roots in the alveolar process is based on the observed fact that as long as the root remains, the bone surrounding it will remain. The support between the denture and the reduced teeth may be a gold coping, a stud attachment, chrome cobalt bearing area, a thimble crown, or the denture may be obtaining some support by merely resting on an amalgam surface of a restored tooth. [19, 35]

Advantages of overdenture

1. The overdenture can resist the occlusal forces better, which are being exerted by mastication in comparison to the completely tissue-borne full denture.

2. Very good support retention and stability can be obtained from the abutment teeth.
3. This overcomes the Old age prosthetic problem of ridge resorption and maintains ridge height. Therefore there is better preservation of vertical dimension.
4. The proprioceptive sensory mechanism derived from the retained roots, is beneficial for the patient. The patients' psychology gets a boost by knowing that he is not totally edentulous. [37]

Disadvantage of overdenture

1. Maximum problems encountered are due to poor case selection and lack of patient cooperation.
2. The teeth under over dentures are prone to caries.
3. In some cases deep gingival pockets are seen to develop around the teeth supporting the dentures. [37]

Indications of overdenture

1. Conditions where it is important to preserve the alveolar ridge and safe guard the ridge from the stress offered by a firm abutment tooth.
2. In case where psychological support provided by overdenture convinces the patient that he or she is not completely edentulous.
3. To preserve vertical dimension.
4. For a partial denture support, an application of overdenture is indicated even if only single abutment is available. [37]

Contraindications

1. Poor alveolar support.
2. An abutment tooth having significant mobility and unmanageable sulcus depth.

3. If the remaining natural teeth are sufficient to restore the mouth with fixed or partial dentures.
4. Those teeth that cannot be retained for long. And those teeth in which it is virtually impossible to develop a sufficient zone of attached gingiva.[37]

SELECTION OF ABUTMENT TEETH

The tooth selected for use as an abutment should be healthy, with significant or minimal mobility. Moreover it should also have an adequate area of attached gingiva, manageable sulcus depth.

Abutment tooth location

1. The ideal teeth to retain are those located where the occlusal forces wreak greatest destruction on the ridges. In natural dentition, the canines are the ideal teeth to retain. In edentulous patients, the anterior area resorbs earlier so canines and premolars are the choice of teeth to be retained. It is important to retain the mandibular teeth because of difficulties encountered in retaining lower dentures.
2. One situation to be warned against however is the diagonal cross arch arrangement – a molar abutment on one side and a canine on the other side. The rocking and torquing action set up by this arrangement leads to problems and loss of one or both abutments. In such cases a molar abutment alone is sufficient.
3. If selected abutment teeth are reduced to round or bullet shape – literally "*tucking*" the abutments inside the denture base – the crown root ratio is vastly improved, especially when periodontally compromised teeth have lost some alveolar support. As shortened teeth, however, they can serve as better abutments for full overdentures.

Procedure

1. After selection of abutment teeth, the teeth to receive root canal fillings are anaesthetized, and a rubber dam is placed.

2. The crowns of these teeth are amputated 3—4 mm above the gingival level.

3. The length of the remaining tooth is established radiographically, and pulps are removed, the canals are shaped and cleaned properly and obturated with guttapercha.

4. The coronal 3—5 mm of filling of guttapercha is then removed, the preparation is undercut, and a well condensed amalgam filling is placed to cap the canal obturation.

5. At this time the abutments should be properly shaped to rise 2—3 mm above the tissue and be round or bullet shaped with a slope back from the labial surface to accommodate the denture tooth set upon it. The abutments should not be too short or the tissue will grow over them as *"lawn growing over a sidewalk"* nor should they be too long, compromising the denture contour and placing greater stress on the supporting teeth. [19]

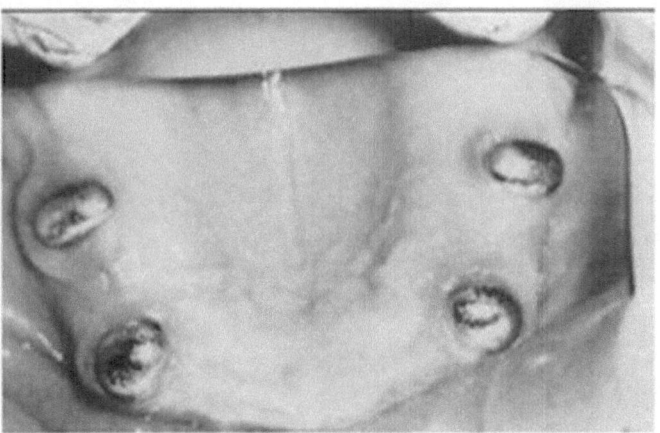

6. The denture is relieved over the abutment until it fits securely on the tissue without touching the abutment teeth. This proper relationship of the denture to the tissue and the tooth is important for denture stability and to keep the stresses on the teeth within physiologic limits.

7. Some teeth are so abraded that pulp has receded to a level where the tooth merely needs shortening, contouring, and polishing.

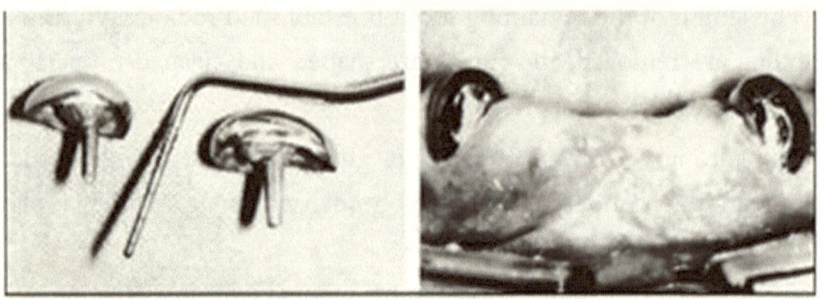

8. If the abutment teeth are involved periodontally or are not supported by a good collar of attached gingiva, periodontal therapy will be needed to correct these aberrations

CONCLUSION AND SUMMARY

- It is very important to remember that in preservation of the endodontically involved or pulpless teeth, the root canal obturation is not the eventual endeavor. Often the success at the apical level is given so much importance, that the coronal destruction gets neglected and not taken care of. If most of the crown is preserved, an anterior tooth can be safely restored with a plastic filling. To guard against the fracture of posterior teeth, cast restorations providing adequate cuspal coverage are recommended. It is important to preserve as much tooth structure as possible, particularly within the root canal, where the amount of dentin remaining may be difficult to assess.
- A post and core is used to provide retention and support for a cast restoration. It should be of adequate length, width, and diameter and should fit properly into the root canals and provide proper apical and coronal seal.
- Anterior teeth are best built up with an esthetic post and core whereas cast metal alloys may be preferred in posterior teeth.
- Due consideration should be given to various restorative and periodontal techniques to protect the fractured tooth which previously was not restored properly.

All the accessible techniques and procedures should be well thought out to restore the tooth properly with the permanence that is due.

REVIEW OF LITERATURE

RAIDEN G. C, H. GENDELMAN (1994)[25]

The aim of this study was to study the effect of post preparation on the apical seal of root fillings. All the specimens were prepared and filled using guttapercha. The guttapercha was then removed leaving different lengths of residual filling material in the canals and a negative control group was also prepared (that is to say filled canals where no dowel space was prepared). After setting the specimens were immersed in a 2% methylene blue dye solution for three days. It was noted that the final length of the apical fillings was found to be different from the intended length in all teeth. As far as leakage was concerned it did not show a significant difference when compared to the control group. In teeth where the maximum length of residual filling material was there showed zero leakage values. These findings may be of clinical importance while restoring short roots.

L. STOCKTON, C.L.B. LAVELLE, M. SUZUKI (1998)[34]

This article discusses that the variations in the utilization of posts to improve the retention of crowns or other restorations on endodontically treated teeth are no longer acceptable now. This practice ignores not only the potential for root perforations during post space preparations, but also the adhesive properties of modern resin-based materials. Since the retention of restorations hinges on many other factors, the placement of posts does not necessarily assure service quality and may even lead to deleterious changes.

The need to reappraise the utilization of posts in the restoration of endodontically treated teeth cannot be overstated.

ANTHONY G. GEGAUFF (2000)[1]

The author has determined the combined effect of crown lengthening and placement of a ferrule on the failure resistance to static load of decoronated and restored mandibular second premolar analog teeth. Ten specimens were prepared with no ferrule root and negligible axial wall lengths and ten specimens with ferrule root, apically repositioned finish lines were made. They were all restored using cast gold alloy posts and cores and complete crowns. Mean failure loads for the crown lengthened / ferrule and no crown lengthened/ no ferrule groups were calculated. He concluded that the combination of simulated crown lengthening and more apical crown margin placement to provide a 2mm crown ferrule on a decoronated mandibular premolar analog resulted in a reduction of static load failure for the restored tooth.

BRETT I. COHEN, MARK K. PAGNILLO, IRA NEWMAN (2000)[6]

The aim of this in vitro study was to compare the retention of two types of core build-up materials (titanium reinforced composite and a GC Miracle Mix silver-reinforced glass ionomer) supported by three post head designs; Flexi-Post, AccessPost, Cerapost dowel.

After the study they concluded that post head designs of the stainless steel AccessPost and Flexi-Post dowels offers greater retention than the smooth ceramic head design of the Cerapost dowel. In addition, the composite core material offers greater retentive strength values than the glass ionomer materials.

BAPANAIAH PANUGONDA, ALLAN SCHULMAN, EUGENE HITTELMAN, BRETT I. COHEN (2000)[2]

This study investigated the effects of post design on the torsional resistance of a crown supported by a titanium reinforced composite core material and three endodontic posts (AccessPost, Flexi-Post, Parapost).

Access Post had the highest torsional value followed by Flexi-Post and Parapost. It was concluded that post design has an effect on torsional resistance of a crown supported by titanium reinforced crown buildup and post. The threaded split shank design of the Flexi-Post dowel offers significantly greater resistance to torsional loading than passive posts studied.

LUIZ NARCISO BARATIERI, MAURO AMARAL CALDEIRA DE ANDRADA, ANDRÉ V. RITTER (2000)[22]

This in vitro study evaluated whether (1) Veneer preparation in enamel or in dentin weakens endodontically treated maxillary incisors; (2) Bonding of direct composite veneer restores the original strength of the unprepared teeth; (3) Use of prefabricated posts increases fracture resistance of prepared and restored teeth.

It was concluded that conservative veneer preparations involving enamel or dentin did not significantly reduce the fracture resistance of endodontically treated maxillary incisors. In addition, restoration of the interenamel preparations with direct composite resulted in teeth more resistant to fracture than teeth having restorations in dentin. The use of posts did not improve the fracture resistance of endodontically treated maxillary incisors reduced and veneered with direct composite.

MARCO FERRARI, ALESSANDRO VICHI, SIMONE GRANDINI, CECILIA GORACCI (2001)[23]

The aim of this study was to evaluate the efficacy of a new bonding luting system in resin tag, adhesive lateral branch, and hybrid layer formation when used in combination with a fiber post. Samples were randomly divided into three groups: Excite light cure bonding agent in combination with Vairolink II resin cement; Excite dual-cured bonding agent self activated by an experimental microbrush in combination with MultiLink resin cement; one step bonding system in combination with Dual Link resin cement.

It was concluded that the dual cure self activating system showed a more uniform resin tag and resin-dentin interdiffusion zone formation along root canal walls than light-curing systems.

STEVEN A. AQUILINO, DANIEL J. CAPLAN (2002)[33]

This study tested the hypothesis that crown placement (coronal coverage) is associated with improved survival of endodontically treated teeth when preaccess, endodontic and restorative factors are controlled. A simple random sample of 280 patients was selected and their dental charts, radiographs, and computerized database were examined to ascertain variables of interest and to verify study inclusion criteria. The results showed that endodontically treated teeth not crowned after obturation were lost at a 6.0 times greater rate than teeth crowned after obturation. Hence they concluded that there is a strong association between crown placement and the survival of endodontically treated teeth.

GUIDO HEYDECKE, MATHILDE C. PETERS (2002)[15]

The aim of this study was to compare the clinical in vitro performance of cast posts and cores to that of direct cores with prefabricated posts in single rooted teeth. Research on the restoration of endodontically treated teeth was identified through a search of electronic databases. This search yielded a total of 1773 references. After these references were subjected to strict inclusion criteria, 10 in vitro and 6 in vivo studies remained and were critically reviewed. A comparison of the fracture loads in the in vitro studies revealed no significant difference between cast and direct posts and cores. Meta analysis of the data suggested that there is no difference in fracture behavior associated with the two treatment modalities. The survival for cast posts and cores in two studies ranged from 87.2% to 88.1% and in third study reached 86.4% for direct cores after 72 months. Randomized clinical trials on this topic were not available but should be conducted to verify published findings.

FRANCESCO MANNOCCI, EGIDIO BERTELLI, MARTYN SHERRIFF, TIMOTHY F. WATSON (2002)[12]

They carried out a study; the aim of which was to evaluate the clinical success rate of endodontically treated premolars restored with fiber posts and direct composite restorations and compare that treatment with a similar treatment of full coverage with metal ceramic crowns. Subjects were randomly assigned to one of the two experimental groups. These studies showed no failures at the one year recall. The only failure reported at two and three years was decementation of posts and clinical or radiographic evidence of marginal gap between tooth and restoration. There was no significant difference in the failure frequencies of the two groups. Hence they concluded that the clinical success rates of endodontically treated teeth restored with fiber posts and direct composite restorations after three years of service were equivalent to a similar treatment to full coverage with metal ceramic crowns.

RAPHAEL PILO, HAROLD S. CARDASH, ELI LEVIN, DAVID ASSIF (2002)[26]

They conducted an in vitro study to examine the effect of core stiffness on the fracture resistance and failure characteristics of a crowned, endodontically treated tooth under simulated occlusal load. Samples were restored using cast post and core, cast crown; preformed metal post, composite core, cast crown; preformed metal post, amalgam core, cast crown; preformed metal post, no core, cast crown. The results did not show any significant difference between the failure load values amongst the four groups. It was concluded that core stiffness did not affect the failure resistance of teeth restored with posts and cores and complete crown coverage cast metal crowns. The dominant pattern of failure was unrepairable root fracture. Only the composite core exhibited repairable fractures.

SEUNG-MI JEONG, KLAUS LUDWIG, MATTHIAS KERN (2002)[30]

The aim of this study was to investigate the fracture resistance of three types of zirconia posts in all ceramic post and core restorations. Three different methods used to fabricate all ceramic post and core restorations: pressing IPS Empress cores directly to zirconia posts; adhesively luting IPS Empress cores to zirconia posts; Celay milling In-Ceram zirconia blanks to one piece post and core restorations.

The highest breaking load and the highest deflection were recorded for the luting technique followed by the pressed cores and the milled zirconia cores. These differences were statistically significant. Regarding the load dependence of the deflection, the luted cores again demonstrated the highest value followed again by pressed-on and milled cores. These differences were not statistically significant. It was concluded that adhesively luted all ceramic cores on zirconia posts offer a viable alternative to the conventional pressed technique.

BEGÜM AKKAYAN, TURGUT GÜLMEZ (2002)[3]

This in vitro study was done to compare the effect of single titanium and three esthetic post systems (quartz fiber posts, glass fiber posts and zirconia posts) on the fracture resistance and fracture patterns of crowned endodontically treated teeth. The results showed that teeth restored with quartz fiber posts exhibited significantly higher resistance to fracture than the other three posts. Teeth restored with glass fiber and zirconia posts were statistically similar. Fractures that would allow repair of the tooth were seen in quartz fiber and glass fiber posts, whereas unrestorable, catastrophic fractures were observed where titanium and zirconia posts were used. Within the limitations of this study, significantly higher failure loads were recorded for root canal treated teeth restores with quartz fiber posts. Fractures that would allow repeated repair were seen with usage of quartz fiber and glass fiber posts.

FRANKLIN R. TAY, SIMONE GRANDINI, CECILIA GORACCI, ROMANO GRANDINI (2005)[31]

The aim of the present study was to present a preliminary clinical report on the use of fiber posts and direct resin composites for restoring root canal treated teeth. The posts used were translucent fiber posts, bonded to the post space using a one-bottle adhesive and dual-cure resin cement.

It was concluded that restoration of endodontically treated teeth with fiber posts and direct resin composites is a treatment option that in the short term conserves remaining tooth structure and results in good patient compliance.

NICO H. J. CREUGERS, ARNO G.M. MENTINK, CEES M. KREULEN (2005)[24]

These studies tested whether the survival rate of cast post and core restorations is better than the survival of direct post and core restorations and post free all composite cores and the survival of these build up restorations is influenced by the remaining dentin height after preparation. These restorations were carried out on patients and treatments were allocated and failures were registered. They found that fifteen restorations failed during the follow up period. Five failures occurred during the first month they were considered to be independent from clinical aging and excluded from further survival accessories. The overall survival was 96% +/- 2%. The factor "remaining dentin heights" appeared to have significant effect of the survival of post and core restorations. They concluded that the type of post and core was not relevant with respect to survival. The amount of remaining dentin height after preparation influenced the longevity of a post and core restoration.

ERICA C.N TEIXEIRA, FABRICIO B. TEIXEIRA, JEFFERY R. PIASICK (2006)[9]

They conducted an in vitro study to characterize the retention, fracture and light transmission behavior of four different fiber reinforced resin-based composite root canal posts. The specimens were divided into four groups according to the types of posts they would receive, that is, parallel fiberglass posts, double tapered fiber quartz posts, tapered fiberglass posts and two different types of parallel fiberglass posts, which were cemented into prepared teeth with dual cured resin cement. They concluded that both tapered posts showed lower retention than the parallel posts and the cement adhered more to the parallel posts than to the tapered posts. All posts showed some plastic behavior, with the double tapered fiberglass post being the stiffest. Translucent prefabricated posts have limited light transmission.

JEFFERSON RICARDO PEREIRA, FABIO DE ORNELAS, PAULO CESAR RODRIGUES CONTI (2006)[18]

The purpose of this study was to compare the fracture strength of endodontically treated teeth using posts and cores and variable quantities of dentin located apical to the core foundations with corresponding ferrule designs incorporated into cast restorations. Sample were divided into four groups and restored and the fracture resistance measured. Significant differences were found among the mean fracture forces of the groups. The mode of failure was recorded as root fracture and the failure in the group with no ferrule occurred due to core fracture, some failures also occurred due to crown cementation failure. They concluded that an increased amount of coronal dentin significantly increases the fracture resistance of endodontically treated teeth.

KERSTIN BITTER, KARSTEN PRIEHN, PETER MARTUS, ANDREJ M. KIELBASSA (2006)[21]

This study initially evaluated the effects of various pretreatment procedures on bond strengths to zirconium-oxide posts using phosphate-methacrylate resin luting agent. Following that investigation, the bond strengths of various luting agents to tribochemically coated glass fiber-reinforced composite resin and zirconium-oxide posts were investigated.

The results showed that bond strengths to the posts were significantly affected by the type of luting agent and type of post. Bond strengths of all luting agents to FRC posts were significantly higher than to the zirconium-oxide posts. Pretreatment procedures significantly increased the bond strength of phosphate-methacrylate resin luting agent to the zirconium-oxide posts. It was concluded that bond strengths of tooth colored posts were significantly affected by the type of luting agent and the type of post and all pretreatment procedures of zirconium-oxide posts significantly increased the bond strength of phosphate-methacrylate resin luting agent.

BIANCA E. M. PEREZ, SILVIA H. BARBOSA, RENATA M. MELO, MARCO A. BOTTINO (2006)[5]

This study aimed to evaluate the influence of cement thickness on the bond strength of a fiber-reinforced composite post system to the root dentin. Samples were randomly divided into two groups and root canals were prepared.

Bond strengths of samples having high and low cement thickness did not show significant difference. But the cement thickness for these groups was significantly different. The increase in cement thickness did not significantly affect the bond strength. Increased cement thickness surrounding the FRC post did not impair the bond strength.

FILIZ AYKENT, MUSTAFA KALKAN, ATILLA GOKHAN OZYESIL (2006)[11]

The aim of this study was to evaluate the effects of two dentin bonding agents and a ferrule preparation on the fracture resistance of crowned mandibular premolars incorporating prefabricated dowels and silver amalgam cores. Samples were divided into six groups and analyzed.

It was observed in the study that, higher fracture strength values were demonstrated for teeth restored with a ferrule and a dual polymerizing resin, followed by those restored with a ferrule and an autopolymerising adhesive, then those restored with only a ferrule with no bonding agent.

A ferrule preparation or a bonding agent designed for silver amalgam core-dentin bonding can each increase the fracture strength for teeth receiving cast crowns after endodontic therapy and dowel and amalgam core restorations.

Bibliography

1. Anthony G. Gegauff; Effect of crown lengthening and ferrule placement on static load failure of cemented cast post cores and crowns. *Journal of Prosthetic Dentistry 2000; vol-84; page no. 169-179.*
2. Bapanaiah Penugonda, Allan Schulman, Eugene Hittelman, Brett I. Cohen; Torsional resistance of crowns cemented to composite cores involving three stainless steel endodontic post designs. *Journal of Prosthetic Dentistry 2000; vol-84; page no. 38-42.*
3. Begum Akkayan, Turgut Gülmez; Resistance to fracture of endodontically treated teeth restored with different post systems. *Journal of Prosthetic Dentistry 2002; vol-87; page no. 431-437.*
4. Bernard G. N. Smith, Leslie C. Home; Planning and Making Crowns and Bridges. *4th edition.*
5. Bianca E. M. Perez, Silvia H. Barbosa, Renata M. Melo, Marco A. Bottino; Does the thickness of the resin cement affect the bond strength of a fiber post to the root dentin? *International Journal of Prosthodontics 2006; vol-19; page no. 606-609.*
6. Brett I. Cohen, Mark K. Pagnillo, Ira Newman; Retention of a core material supported by three post head designs. *Journal of Prosthetic Dentistry 2000; vol-83; page no. 624-628.*
7. Cavazos Jr., Malone, Koth, Kaiser; Tylman's Theory and Practice of Fixed Prosthodontics. *8th edition.*
8. Christopher J. R. Stock, Gulabivala, Richard T. Walker; Endodontics. *2nd edition.*

9. Erica C.N Teixeira, Fabricio B. Teixeira, Jeffery R. Piasick; An in vitro assessment of prefabricated fiber post systems. *Journal of American Dental Association 2006; vol-137; page no. 1006-1012.*

10. Fenn Liddelow and Gimson; Clinical Dental Prosthetics. *3rd edition.*

11. Filiz Aykent, Mustafa Kalkan, Atilla Gokhan Ozyesil; Effect of dentin bonding and ferrule preparation on the fracture strength of crowned teeth restored with dowels and amalgam cores. *Journal of Prosthetic Dentistry 2006; vol-95; page no. 297-301.*

12. Francesco Mannocci, Egidio Bertelli, Martyn Sherriff, Timothy F. Watson; Three year clinical comparison of survival of endodontically treated teeth restored with either full cast coverage or with direct composite restoration. *Journal of Prosthetic Dentistry 2002; vol-88; page no. 297-301.*

13. Franklin S. Weine; Endodontic Therapy. *5th edition.*

14. Graham J. Mount, W.R. Hume; Preservation and Conservation of Tooth Structure. *1st edition.*

15. Guido Heydecke, Mathilde C. Peters; The restoration of endodontically treated, single rooted teeth with cast or direct posts and cores: A systematic review. *Journal of Prosthetic Dentistry 2002; vol-87; page no. 380-386.*

16. Guttman, Dumsha, Lovdhal; Problem Solving in Endodontics – Prevention, Identification and Management. *4th edition.*

17. Harty's; Endodontics in Clinical Practice. *4th edition.*

18. Jefferson Ricardo Pereira, Fabio de Ornelas, Paulo Cesar Rodrigues Conti; Effect of a crown ferrule on the fracture resistance of endodontically treated teeth restored with prefabricated posts. *Journal of Prosthetic Dentistry 2006; vol-95; page no. 50-54.*

19. John I. Ingle, Leif Bakland; Endodontics. *5th edition.*

20. Kenneth M. Hargreaves, Steven Cohen; Pathways of the Pulp. *9th edition.*

21. Kerstin Bitter, Karsten Priehn, Peter Martus, Andrej M. Kielbassa; In vitro evaluation of push-out bond strengths of various luting agents to tooth colored posts. *Journal of Prosthetic Dentistry 2006; vol-95; page no. 302-310.*

22. Luiz Narciso Baratieri, Mauro Amaral Caldeira de Andrada, André V. Ritter; Influence of post placement in the fracture resistance of endodontically treated incisors veneered with direct composite. *Journal of Prosthetic Dentistry 2000; vol-84; page no. 180-184.*

23. Marco Ferrari, Alessandro Vichi, Simone Grandini, Cecilia Goracci; Efficacy of a self-curing adhesive-resin system on luting glass-fiber posts into root canals: **An SEM investigation.** *International Journal of Prosthodontics 2001; vol-14; page no. 543-549.*

24. Nico H. J. Creugers, Arno G.M. Mentink, Cees M. Kreulen; Five year follow-up of a prospective clinical study on various types of core restorations. *International Journal of Prosthodontics 2005; vol-18; page no. 34-39.*

25. Raiden G. C, H. Gendelman; Effect of dowel space preparation on the apical seal of root fillings. *Endodontics and Dental Traumatology 1994; vol-10; page no. 109-112.*

26. Raphael Pilo, Harold S. Cardash, Eli Levin, David Assif; Effect of core stiffness on the in vitro fracture of crowned, endodontically treated teeth. *Journal of Prosthetic Dentistry 2002; vol-38; page no. 302-306.*

27. Ronand E. Goldstein; Esthetics in Dentistry. *2nd edition.*

28. Satish Chandra, Shaleen Chandra; Textbook of Endodontics. *1st edition.*

29. Satish Chandra; Textbook of Operative Dentistry. *1st edition.*

30. Seung-Mi Jeong, Klaus Ludwig, Matthias Kern; Investigation of the fracture resistance of three types of zirconia posts in all-ceramic post and core restorations. *International Journal of Prosthodontics 2002; vol-15; page no. 154-158.*

31. Simone Grandini, Franklin R. Tay, Cecilia Goracci, Romano Grandini; Clinical evaluation of the use of fiber posts ad direct resin restorations for

endodontically treated teeth. ***International Journal of Prosthodontics 2005; vol-18; page no. 399-404.***

32. Stephen F. Rosenstiel, Martin F. Land, Junhei Fujimoto; Contemporary Fixed Prosthodontics. ***2nd edition.***

33. Steven A. Aquilino, Daniel J. Caplan; Relationship between crown placement and the survival of endodontically treated teeth. ***Journal of Prosthetic Dentistry 2002; vol-87; page no. 256-263.***

34. Stockton L. Lavelle, Suzuki M; Are posts mandatory for the restoration of endodontically treated teeth? ***Endodontics and Dental Traumatology 1998; vol-14; page no. 59-63.***

35. Usha Dabas, Vipin K. Dabas; Textbook of Endodontics. **1st edition.**

36. Walton and Torabinejad; Principles and Practice of Endodontics. ***3rd edition.***

37. Zarb and Bolender; Prosthodontic Treatment for Edentulous Patients. ***12th edition.***

www.ingramcontent.com/pod-product-compliance
Lightning Source LLC
Chambersburg PA
CBHW030849180526
45163CB00004B/1508